IØ110001

Praise for
The Dance of Resilience

"This is a powerful testament to dance as a force for resilience and recovery. These stories echo what scientific research increasingly shows: Partner dance improves quality of life. It's an inspiring call for integrating dance into mainstream health and well-being practice."
—DR. PETER LOVATT, dance psychologist and author of *The Dance Cure*

"*The Dance of Resilience* is a powerful testament to how movement changes people. Through shared connection and courage we discover healing, joy, and our deepest strength. This inspiring book beautifully illustrates how dancing with others can lead us back to ourselves."
— BONNIE BURTON, former Regional District Director, USA Dance, Inc.

"*The Dance of Resilience* powerfully reveals how dance boosts brain health and mental well-being. With inspiring stories and compelling science, it makes a clear case: Dance isn't just movement—it's medicine. It's a must-read for anyone passionate about wellness, aging, and community healing."
—WAYNE ENG AND MARIA HANSEN, leaders at Dance Vision Foundation

"*The Dance of Resilience* brilliantly tells the story of the power of ballroom dance and how far-reaching and impactful it is. Health insurance carriers and self-funded employers need to get fully on board with their support and walk the talk. It's the #1 activity that supports brain and physical health!"

— JEANIE LAFAVOR, Vice President of Sales, HealthEZ

"As a physician and musician, I've seen how music and movement can improve brain health and physical well-being. This book is an overdue call to action for policymakers and health leaders to bring prescriptions for dance and other arts into our insured and public health systems to help reduce costs and improve health."

— DR. ALAN SIEGEL, cofounder of Social Prescribing USA

"I firmly believe dance is both a beautiful art form and a fitness pathway for people to get into the best shape of their lives. Ember weaves together heartfelt stories with proven results, creating powerful testimony that dance is both."

— LOUIS VAN AMSTEL, *Dancing with the Stars* professional and founder of LaBlast Fitness

"In my years as a professional competitive dancer and coach, I've not seen a resource like this: remarkable, heartfelt life stories to inspire the beginner or veteran dancer. If this well-written treasure doesn't inspire you to pick up your dance shoes, I don't know what will!"

— JAIMEE TUFT, World and US professional ballroom dance champion

"Ember has woven together a compelling and accessible narrative that highlights the deep, transformative power of dance across diverse communities and health contexts— including the Dance for PD community I help lead. I hope her clear-eyed exploration of dance as an art form and a public health intervention inspires more partnerships between the dance world and the medical community."

—DAVID LEVENTHAL, Program Director,
Dance for PD® at Mark Morris Dance Group

The DANCE *of* RESILIENCE

The DANCE *of* RESILIENCE

**Transforming Lives and Staying Vibrant
Through Partner Dance**

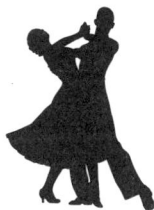

Ember Reichgott Junge

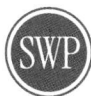

SWP

SHE WRITES PRESS

Published in 2026 by
She Writes Press, an imprint of The Stable Book Group

SWP

32 Court Street, Suite 2109
Brooklyn, NY 11201
https://shewritespress.com
Library of Congress Control Number: 2025915420
ISBN: 979-8-89636-042-1
eISBN: 979-8-89636-043-8

Interior Designer: Tabitha Lahr
Back cover photo: Eliza Doolittle and Henry Higgins showcase *My Fair Lady* (a.k.a Ember Reichgott Junge and ballroom dance instructor Chris Inveen) at Snow Ball DanceSport Competition, 2025; Photo compliments of Dance Production House.

Printed in the United States

This book is dedicated to my mother, Diane Reichgott, the jitterbug queen who produced plays and choreographed dances for me and my schoolmates while planting seeds in my heart and soul that finally took root decades later.

Contents

PART I: Transforming Life Through the Power of Dance

PART II: What's Holding *You* Back?

PART III: Relationships: Breaking Down and Breaking Through—Together

PART IV: Breaking through Gender, Racial, and Cultural Barriers

PART V: Dance Science: Medicine for the Aging Body, Mind, and Soul

PART VI: Call to Action

PART I

Transforming Life through the Power of Dance

The life-changing power of dance is that it helps you discover your hidden resilience. Resilience is about more than surviving difficult circumstances. It's about letting go, giving up control, being vulnerable, listening—even when every part of your being resists. It's about overcoming unreasonable fears.

All this can be discovered—often unexpectedly—through the delight of dance.

Chapter 1

Waltz into Life-Changing Self-Discovery

When I walked into my first ballroom dance studio at the age of thirty-five, I had one purpose in mind—to find a husband. I found one. But he doesn't dance a step unless he drinks five beers.

Dance changed *me*. Dance transformed my life one day at a time.

From all outward signs, I was living a successful and happy life. I was a young attorney and Minnesota state senator, pathways few women pursued in the late 1970s and early '80s.

I thought I was pretty resilient in the face of new challenges, especially those I faced professionally in a man's world. Yes, I was "able to withstand or recover quickly from difficult conditions," as the Oxford Dictionary defines *resilience*.

But I was paying a price. The road was lonely. My authentic self was buried deep inside.

My dance journey slowly opened my eyes. Resilience meant so much more. For me, it meant giving up control. Letting go. Being vulnerable. Listening. Trying something new. Confronting unreasonable fears I'd learned as "truth" from parents, family, and media. Breaking through those fears to self-discovery. Finding the courage to sustain the new shining light in my life. Expressing my satisfaction and pleasure in a whole new way.

Dance helped me become the better, more authentic person I wanted to be. A person who could love myself first—then love another person.

Over the years, I've seen other people grow not only as dancers but also as authentic human beings. I've watched ordinary people overcome extraordinary challenges through the power of partner dance. Their resilience inspired me.

Their stories are the real focus of this book. They reveal in their own words how dance nourished their mind, body, and spirit. As a former journalist, I weave snippets of my personal journey into the immersive experiences of others.

At its core, this book is about much more than dance. It's about personal development, health and wellness, and finding purpose and joy. For every breakdown, there is a breakthrough.

The transformations are remarkable. My own life experience is Exhibit A.

How does this happen? Why are some people willing to jump into the uncertainty and not others? What is it about partner dance, specifically, that breaks down innate fears from childhood and opens a new world of self-discovery? How does dance help people overcome setbacks that seem insurmountable?

I was on a mission to find out for this book. I talked with social dancers, amateur competitors, and teaching professionals, ranging from ten-year-old fifth graders to ninety-three-year-old Angela. These dancers were gay, straight, African American, Russian, Latino, Hmong, and more. Some broke cultural barriers with their passion for dance.

It is my good fortune to personally know or have known each person who shared a story in this book.

There's my dance partner, Dennis, who found dance to be the greatest healer in his recovery from cancer.

There's Lisa, who never let being blind stop her from dancing. And Jim, who ran away from home at fourteen and discovered dance in his fifties—after his thigh had been gored by a buffalo and he'd been told he would never walk again.

There's Paul, a seventy-year-old surgeon who revealed his right-leg prosthesis as he danced an emotional waltz before a packed ballroom.

And Regina, a native of South Korea who discovered dance at age sixty, which helped her restore a shattered self-image after an abusive marriage.

These are all ordinary people like you and me. So how did the discipline, connection, and movement of partner dance unpack years of "I can't" or "I won't" for them? How did partner dance build a self-confidence never experienced before?

Even professional dancers and celebrities start somewhere. Like my dance teacher Nathan, who grew up in the deep South and is now one of only four male African American ballroom dance judges in North America.

Perhaps you are familiar with the Bersten family. The elder Berstens came to Minnesota from the former Soviet Union with only pennies in their pockets, yet their children created a studio filled with nationally reputed dancers. Alan Bersten is a celebrity professional on the hit television show *Dancing with the Stars*.

Finally, who doesn't know Suni Lee, the Olympic-gold-medalist gymnast and *Dancing with the Stars* semifinalist? She and her clan grandmother, a refugee from Laos, put the Hmong culture on the world map and introduced partner dance to the Hmong community.

Talk about resilience!

Dance also builds—and tests—the resilience of marriages and relationships. Dance can reenergize midlife marriage. What *are* those marital secrets? Sometimes long-time life and dance partners realize they can no longer be both. Painful. Grieving spouses turn to dance for social connection, totally outside their comfort zone, leading to new love once again.

And why did it take so long for same-sex partner dance to break through the traditional world of ballroom dance?

There are also joyful stories of transformations for fifth and eighth graders who danced in Dancing Classrooms, a program brought to Minnesota schools by the Heart of Dance nonprofit I co-founded. Take Maya, for example. Suspended in fourth grade for bad behavior, Maya lit up in Dancing Classrooms and became a class leader in fifth grade, to the awe of parents and teachers. What was it about partner dance that broke through that child's wall of resistance?

Perhaps most important is the enormous impact partner dance and dance movement can make in improving quality of life for senior citizens and those living with dementia or Parkinson's disease. Partner dance can reverse symptoms of Parkinson's. And research shows that partner dance is 76 percent more effective in preventing dementia (or delaying its progress) than any other form of exercise.

Let me repeat that: *76 percent!*

How can that be? What is the scientific basis for that? It's real. Yet we don't hear much about it. Why not? What prevents so many seniors from engaging in something so accessible that can bring proven health and social benefits?

That's why I built on these remarkable stories with an urgent Call to Action at the end of the book. We can and *must* bring dance and its proven outcomes into local community services and the traditional insured health care system. The likely result? Thousands of people will live healthier lives, lowering health care costs for all.

As you resonate with these courageous storytellers, take a moment to think about your own story. The themes in this book are universal and real. What in *your* life is holding you back? What is *your* wall of resistance deep inside you? What fulfillment and satisfaction await *you* when you confront your fears, take those first few dance steps, and open your mind and body to a whole new world?

Let go. Be vulnerable. Try something new. Let these story-tellers show you the way. You just don't know what you'll discover for yourself.

Give yourself the greatest gift of all: Explore the Dance of Resilience.

Chapter 2

⌄

My Story:
From First Lesson
to First Performance
to First Love

My whole body was shaking. It was my first dance lesson with young instructor John Abrams of Arthur Murray Dance Studio.

He took my hand. "Can you do this?"

Nervously, I nodded. I moved—and screwed up.

I look like a dork. What does he think of me? I'm so uncoordinated. My mom would laugh at me if she saw this.

I frowned. I moved my foot—and stepped on his toe.

Argh! One, two, three. It shouldn't be this hard. He must think I'm stupid. I've never been able to dance. Why am I doing this? He would never be a candidate for my husband. I think he's gay.

He took my waist.

Don't touch me. I don't want to go there! I just put on five pounds right around the waist.

I just know the other students are staring at me. I wish they would go away. Why can't we be in a room with no other students?

They probably know me as that senator they've seen on television.
I'm so embarrassed! I'm paying good money for this . . . ?
"Side together back," he said.
OK. Side together, forward—ouch!
"I'm so sorry!" I said.
"No worries," he replied. "You just need to relax."
Oh sure. You can *say that—you've been doing this forever.*
There's got *to be a better way to find a husband than this!*

∽◎◌

I had to reach deep inside to find the courage to walk into that dance studio that day. I'd never really danced in my life. In fact, I'd resisted it. I knew I was a lousy dancer, especially compared to my mother, the jitterbug queen and former Arthur Murray instructor. She intimidated the hell out of me. I knew I could never live up to her expectations of me in dance.

But I felt like I had to do something radical. For years, I'd been pretty much married to my careers as a lawyer and a legislator. Intense and driven, I didn't take time to play. I wasn't much fun, and I was growing anxious. My biological clock was ticking, but I wasn't in a relationship.

When I became a career woman in my twenties, I instinctively thought I had to act like a man. I had to be professional. I had to be perfect. God knows I couldn't make a mistake, at least not publicly.

I wore those little ties at the neck, like a man's bow tie. I dressed in matched suits and wore very little jewelry. One reporter described me as "perfectly coiffed." At the time, I thought that was a compliment. Now I realize he was describing my lack of authenticity. Ouch! I was all about "looking good" for my constituents, the media, and whoever else was watching—twenty-four hours a day, seven days a week.

But there was one way I could be me, and it was with music. In college, I performed in musical theater and traveled the world with the international musical group Up with People. In the senate, my best friends were colleagues who played guitars and sang with me after hours. I didn't need alcohol. Music lifted my heart. But I rarely—if ever—danced.

Maybe it was the music that triggered something deep inside me during those first few months of my dance journey. Dance opened my heart and mind and started to heal me in ways I didn't think possible. For the first time, I had a safe place to be me, the *real* me. I could let go. I could make a mistake and be vulnerable. I could laugh at myself and with others. I could explore my femininity and "try on" elegance in movement and in lovely dresses that hugged my body. It felt so good.

And maybe, just maybe, I could be as elegant and confident as my mother, with her beautiful stature and presence.

Fast-forward one year.

Sweat beaded on my forehead as I stood on the edge of the dance floor. In just seconds, I would start my first-ever dance showcase with my professional teacher, John Abrams. We'd been practicing this forty-five-second waltz showcase for nearly a year.

This was a solo performance—just me and my teacher. The other students, teachers, and families all had eyes on me. I wanted—*needed*, more than anything—to dance well because my mother, the former Arthur Murray dance instructor, was in the audience.

John escorted me onto the well-lit dance floor. I walked tall and straight, as he'd taught me. I faced him. The music began.

John extended his arm to invite me to dance. I fought back the panic. It was everything I could do to receive his hand, move into dance frame position, and not turn around and run. I was going to dance—something I never thought I could do! Something I'd always been so self-conscious about.

The soft, lilting notes of the waltz came through. *One, two, three. One, two, three.* I'm sure I was hanging on to John for dear life.

I glanced over my shoulder. There was my mother, beaming. Absolutely beaming. At last, after thirty-five years, her daughter was dancing.

I felt the spotlight all over my body, feeding energy to every cell. John twirled me. My nearly calf-length black dress with silver trim swirled about my legs. I felt like an elegant princess.

I smelled the familiar scent of my teacher's cologne. I smiled, feeling safe with him. I let my body fall into the music. *Pivot, one, two, three.* It was happening!

I stretched my arm out to the audience, right toward my mother. I smiled at her over my extended arm.

The music crescendoed as John brought me into his arms and dipped me to the ground to end the dance.

It was the longest—and shortest—forty-five seconds of my dance career. I heard the applause. I saw the tears in my mother's eyes.

Tears welled up in my own eyes. I did it! I'd danced a beautiful waltz. No panic. Just sheer exhilaration! A new world had opened up for me.

I bowed, as I'd been taught. John escorted me off the floor, with me smiling and tears falling down my face.

I rushed over to my mother. We hugged and hugged. I knew I'd exceeded her expectations.

I could do this! And I would do it again. And again.

❧

As I learned new dance steps, my confidence grew. I discovered the child within me and the pure fun that went with it. I forgot the state budget and the worries of the world when I was on the dance floor.

I could safely touch a man without worrying about his intentions. I could be more comfortable and trusting around multiple male dance partners. I could laugh with them, relax and enjoy them, and not worry about whether they liked me or thought me attractive. I could just focus on the beauty and precision of the movement, the beat of the music, and the dance picture we were creating together.

This world was so unlike the legislature, where I believed women had to be stoic, professional, and nearly perfect. And where women might be approached by male lobbyists and colleagues with sexual intentions to yield desired legislative outcomes.

I discovered my authentic self, which had been hidden for so long. I became a person full of life. I could be myself. I could love myself.

And I could love Mike, my future husband, when he entered my life four years after I walked into that dance studio. I don't think I would have opened my heart to him without first opening myself to ballroom dance.

When Mike called me for our second date, I had a dance showcase that night. Would he come? He agreed. I guess you'll do anything for a date if you're interested enough.

That was the first and nearly last time Mike would watch me dance. It wasn't his thing. So we made a bargain for our wedding day—I wouldn't teach Mike to dance, and he wouldn't teach me to golf.

Fast-forward to today: We've been happily married for over thirty years. My plan worked—but in many more ways than I'd ever imagined, as I'll share in coming chapters.

Yes, ballroom dance transformed my life, one step at a time. It had a profound impact on me. That said, the impact it had on me doesn't come close to the impact it had on some of my dancer friends. They had remarkable experiences. Remarkable life changes. Remarkable resilience. Remarkable heartfelt stories.

Dennis is one of those dancers. He will take us next on one man's journey through the healing power of ballroom dance.

Chapter 3

⌣

The Greatest
Therapy of All

Dennis Yelkin felt broken. He'd been nauseated for six weeks after receiving a powerful chemo blast to treat his multiple myeloma in June 2018. His life was on hold; his world was small. He lay in bed. *One more breath. Don't throw up.* He was back to his "loner" days, just like he'd experienced as a teen and young adult.

"When I'm sick, I'm my own best caregiver," he said. "I don't need anyone. Visitors are an intrusion to my privacy."

Dennis was all alone, except for his life partner, Jim.

I was one of the few visitors Dennis allowed. As his social dance partner, I did my best to provide support. I could hardly know what Dennis was going through, though. Mostly, we talked about our longing to dance again.

That wouldn't happen until months later, at our December Social Dance Club black-tie dinner.

"I was so happy I could dance again and see people," Dennis said. "Life was going to be OK. I was getting my appetite back.

But could I even do it? I think muscle memory took over. So many things to think about—dance steps, rhythm, synchronizations. They happen quicker than you can think. There are constant impulses and strategies. It's wonderful mind-body therapy. I craved the physical contact. I missed it so much."

Dennis wore his wool tuxedo, which hung loosely on his thin frame, and his gray knit chemo hat. We celebrated as we danced waltz and rumba to live music. Dennis was back, at least physically. Our friends welcomed him.

At my urging, he asked my college friend Barbara Peterson Burwell (a former Miss USA) to dance. They looked elegant together. He didn't know that Barbara's husband had battled multiple myeloma before he died, or that Barbara was a cancer survivor herself.

As Dennis recalled:

I casually told Barbara I was warm in my wool tux and cancer cap to cover my peach fuzz.

"Why don't you take the cap off?" she asked.

"Oh, I'd be embarrassed."

"Why would you be embarrassed? You're among friends."

I realized at that moment that I was among friends, and that I would be more comfortable being my true self, which was peach-fuzz head.

I took off my hat. Such relief! My head was sweating. I focused on dancing with Barbara. I wanted to make her look good. People told me I looked great. They told me I had a nice-shaped head.

That night was the beginning of my real recovery . . . my emotional recovery. I felt new energy. I got so much positive feedback that it gave me confidence. It was just a relief to not have that damn hat on around other people.

OK, I can do this. People are fine with it.

In the coming days, I saw Dennis's transformation firsthand. As he gained strength, I suggested we do something new—create a dance routine to track our journey together through his painful health challenge.

He was hesitant at first. We asked dance professional Scott Anderson to choreograph it. Scott's wife selected Carole King's "You've Got a Friend" as a musical message from me.

"Because of our long working relationships, we were candid with each other if something didn't work," Dennis said. "In the end, the process of creating that routine was the best therapy I could have had."

The routine evolved over a year. It started with a depressed Dennis in his chemo cap.

"When I stooped over at the beginning of the routine, it was authentic," he recalled. "I felt broken, even though my lab numbers were getting better. Scott, in his genius, helped me portray how I felt after that cancer blast."

As for me, I learned ways to visibly encourage Dennis back to dance, even lifting his arm onto my shoulder to partner.

We both knew what came next—I needed to remove his cap to free him.

"When you pulled my cancer cap off during the routine, I had a visceral, gut reaction because that hat was what I was hiding behind," Dennis admitted. "I didn't want to talk to people about my health, yet I was wearing the emblem of cancer. I hated that hat, but it was my security blanket. So, when I desperately reached out for that hat during our routine, it was from the gut."

From there, joy emerged, and Dennis grew stronger. He dipped me; we celebrated. He lifted me.

What? A lift?

When Scott first suggested a lift, I wasn't so sure. Dennis was trained in dance improvisation, but he was then seventy-four years old, was slowly gaining weight from a low of 137 pounds, and was still recovering from cancer. I was only a few years younger and not exactly petite. We were solid midlevel competitive dancers, but certainly not dance champions.

Really? A lift?

The courage Dennis had! Sure, we had a fall along the way, in an early performance. But with Scott's help, we found a lift that worked.

"When I lifted you up and spun you around—I was celebrating!" Dennis exclaimed. "I was flying! It was a big . . . *YES!*"

We kept at it. As Dennis shared, "Very often during rehearsals, we both got teary eyed because it brought back memories of when I was so sick. It was difficult to demonstrate to Scott or others how vulnerable I was. When I was sick, I thought I didn't need anyone. But during this routine, I realized that I *did* need other people's help, and that's one reason I got emotional. I realized *how much* I needed other people—something I'd never admitted to myself."

Dance, I realized, can widen our self-perceptions.

"A person can go to a private therapist or group therapy," Dennis said. "But to visually and viscerally tell our story through dance was the type of therapy and healing I needed. I didn't want to go around talking to everybody. I was able to physically express what I felt. Who gets to do this if they're not in the dance world? Dancing is such a significant and powerful way to tell a story that words could never express."

Dennis was declared in remission in September 2019. At the same time, and by coincidence, competition organizer Donna Edelstein was creating a special "Cancer Conquerors" focus for the January 2020 competitors. A recent cancer survivor herself, Donna invited Dennis and me to showcase our routine on the final evening.

We danced with everything we had. The performance was our best.

"We reacted to each other's emotions authentically," Dennis said. "They were real. That's what the audience felt. I never danced anything like that before."

Nor had I. It felt good. We fed off each other in our friendship and bond of over twenty-eight years.

As one judge critiqued, "I can see—it's being danced from the soul."

From another: "Such a powerfully emotional solo. Thank you."

Dennis, the self-described loner in his early years, was his authentic adult self—a connector. That night, he connected hearts with strangers and love with friends. So many friends. He inspired other cancer survivors. Some rose to their feet.

It was the healing power of dance. The greatest therapy of all.

Chapter 4

❦

I'm Not Going to Live in God's Waiting Room

I originally wrote this story in 2022, when Roger and Melinda Martin were seventy-four. But in 2023, they both earned their angel wings, passing away just twelve weeks apart—Roger on March 23, and Melinda on June 13. I've preserved the story as I wrote it, so that it might celebrate their lives.

Roger and Melinda Martin, both seventy-four, know they don't have much time left. But they don't live in that mind-set. They keep going. They always plan for more things to do—mainly dance and travel.

Melinda has lived with terminal heart failure for fifteen years. She "died" twice but was resuscitated. The first time was on the ballroom dance floor in 2008. (Stay tuned for more on that story.)

Since 2018, Melinda has worn a fifteen-pound left ventricular assist device (LVAD), a piece of electrical equipment that keeps her heart going. That's the only way she stays alive. But it means she can't fit into her beloved dance dresses or dance Halloween costumes any longer. Today, her dancewear must allow room for the special vest that's filled with metal components, tubes, and wires.

And that will never change. An LVAD is normally only used as a bridge for a person waiting for a heart transplant. But Melinda's body isn't eligible for a transplant, so the LVAD is her only option.

She's lived a difficult, painful, exhausting, and limited life. But as she said, "You make it a good life."

Roger's life isn't easy either. He's recovering from stage II pancreatic cancer, diagnosed in the summer of 2021. He lost significant weight during his chemotherapy and subsequent surgery. And here in the fall of 2022, he's functioning at only half his normal energy level. But the good news is that he's cancer-free and has a good shot at "a few more years."

"A miracle!" Melinda declared.

Roger and Melinda will take this miracle and every day it provides them. They understand the odds: With a stage II diagnosis, pancreatic cancer always comes back.

What's so remarkable about this couple is that they've maintained their dance-lesson schedule as best as they can, despite all these years of Melinda's severe medical trauma and Roger's more recent diagnosis. They've also continued to travel on yearly dance trips whenever possible.

"We were driven through this to dance and travel," said Roger. "And that certainly provided the drive, especially for Melinda, whose love of dance is unmatched. I think it provided her a pathway to navigate and negotiate all of this shit!"

Their travel won't stop anytime soon either. "I'm not going to stop planning because we are going to die," said Melinda. "We're both dying. There's no question about that. But I have three cruises booked, paid for, and planned. I have no intention of canceling—unless I need to on the very last day. We won't have anything if we don't plan. I'm not going to live in God's waiting room. I'm going to go out and play. And dance and play, whether I breathe well or not."

The couple is grateful to have the financial resources to do this. "We're using them in a way we never planned because we know both of us are terminal," Melinda explained. "We don't need a certain amount of income from our portfolio every month until we are a hundred and one. So we changed the way we use our portfolio. We gave ourselves the means to travel in a way we need to, which is first-class. On a cruise ship, we need a large suite because of the LVAD. I need space. I need room. I don't fit anywhere but first-class with all the equipment I have to wear."

‿❦⁀

Roger and Melinda have been dancing together since the first day they met, when they were computer-matched as University of Minnesota freshmen during Welcome Week. Their first dance was to "Moon River" on September 22, 1966. They married in June 1970, upon graduation.

They continued to dance freestyle for many years. Around 1999, with just one of two children still at home, Roger initiated the "gift to ourselves" to take ballroom dance lessons at Dancers Studio in Saint Paul. Melinda's younger brother, Glen Lindgren, was a student at the studio, having started ballroom dance years before in the University of Minnesota Dance Club.

"We'd talked casually about learning ballroom dance for years," Roger said. "So I just decided to follow up on it. I wanted to act on the dream we'd discussed between us many times."

The couple loved their dance lessons. Dance brought relief after their many working hours. Roger ran a consulting engineering business, and Melinda was a school media specialist and librarian.

And while they didn't compete themselves, they attended the Twin Cities Open (TCO) competition each year to support their studio friends. It was at TCO in Bloomington, Minnesota, on July 11, 2008, that Melinda first learned she had health issues. That night, she and Roger danced four times during the general dances, then they stood to the side to cheer on their friends getting ready for the formation team competition.

Without warning, Melinda fell to the floor.

"I simply dropped dead," she said. "I had ventricular fibrillation, which is sudden death for a heart. You don't survive this whether you're in a hospital or not."

Melinda's brother was there and started the breathing side of CPR. A medical student from Dancers Studio jumped into action with chest compressions. Someone called 911, sending EMTs on the way.

In the first of several miracles, the ensemble of dancers on the floor just happened to consist of eight physicians and nurses from Mayo Clinic in Rochester, Minnesota. They ran top-speed diagonally across the huge ballroom floor at the (then) Radisson South Hotel to step in with the CPR.

The medical team continued CPR as they waited for the EMTs to arrive. But they never once got a sign of life.

There was no sign of life from Melinda for nine minutes and forty-six seconds.

When the EMTs at last arrived, they made two hits with a defibrillator. At last, a breath and a heartbeat.

"Those doctors and nurses never stopped—they never stopped the blood flowing," Melinda said. "Since I actually did come back to life, I didn't have brain damage or heart damage. That was solely because of their quick efforts."

Roger continued, "The nurses at the hospital told us that the chance of surviving what Melinda experienced is less than 1 percent—and that's for people who are already in the hospital. You're looking at a miracle. It just doesn't happen."

Prior to the ventricular fibrillation, Melinda had experienced good health, without a "hint of anything" troublesome. Doctors eventually discovered that she had a virus in her body from when she was a child. She had been born in Japan and raised in Germany. The virus had caused a cold that decimated her body and left her with a very weak heart, though she'd experienced no symptoms before. Surgeons fit Melinda with a defibrillator that would shock her heart back to life if it happened again.

As it turned out, that virus was just getting started wreaking havoc in Melinda's body. Just three years later, she was diagnosed with breast cancer, forcing her to quit her job. She also had seven surgeries for skin cancer.

Then in 2016, the breast cancer reoccurred, resulting in a double mastectomy. That same year, Melinda had massive surgery for a condition known as Type III achalasia of the esophagus plus failure of a valve that allows food into the stomach. All caused by the virus.

To make matters worse, the latter surgery was delayed because she was in a back brace for five months, recovering from a smashed vertebrae that occurred while dancing with Roger on a dance trip to Puerto Vallarta.

Finally, in 2019, Melinda's heart gave out a second time, resulting in the difficult decision to implant the LVAD for the rest of her life. The virus prevented her from becoming eligible for a heart transplant.

～◎～

Through all this, Melinda continued to dance.

"I can dance through anything," she said with a smile. "The way Mayo Clinic put it is that you create your own wellness. I made sure I did everything to be as well as I could so I could keep dancing."

How did she do that?

"I don't know," she admitted. "You just do it. Your life changes—not just as a person but as a couple—when you die and come back. I had to retire early. To me, then, that was the beginning for Roger and me to make significant changes and to add significant wonderful things to our life. Dancing and travel. Like a bucket list. I finished that bucket list."

One change they made was to celebrate milestones early and often. While many couples celebrate their fiftieth wedding anniversaries, Melinda and Roger decided to pull out all the stops for their fortieth anniversary in 2010.

They decided to dance their first-ever showcase at the celebration, to the music of their first dance, "Moon River." They spent eight months working on a waltz routine at the Silver (intermediate) level with instructor Jill Johnson.

"We nailed it to perfection," Roger exulted. "Every move of every part of our body was choreographed and practiced again and again for eight months."

"It was wonderful!" Melinda agreed.

"It was one of the most exhilarating experiences I've ever had," Roger admitted. "We're both complete perfectionists. Jill told us she was trying to bring us down to reality and that we would have a glitch or a bobble. We didn't. It was perfect."

Melinda did live to their fiftieth anniversary in 2020, but she wouldn't have been able to do that waltz showcase. With the LVAD, Roger had to dance differently with her. There were moves they couldn't do any longer.

"We've learned how to adapt all the way through my heart failure, with much help from instructors," said Melinda. "You adapt and you pace, you adapt and you pace, because of my breathing. It's almost like learning to dance all over again. My biggest problem besides fatigue and chest pains is shortness of breath."

Talk about resilience.

Both spouses are dancing their way through their terminal health journeys. And they will keep dancing until the end. Something tells me they'll revisit that perfect fortieth anniversary waltz routine in the future—with angel wings to guide them.

❧

Indeed, they danced until their end on this earth. I'd love to see their new heavenly dance routines.

Chapter 5

〜

You'll Never Walk Again

Jim Carter ran away from home at age fourteen. He never went to high school. He hated school in part because his family moved around, causing him to attend seven different schools in seven states over the course of only one year.

Jim's dad was an alcoholic who abused his mom. At age twelve, Jim discovered that alcohol worked for him as well. Within a few years, he became a full-blown alcoholic. By age nineteen, Jim didn't care about anything. He hitchhiked across the United States and Canada to Alaska, working day jobs along the way.

"I was the kid off the street," he said. "I should have been in jail. I was an angry young man. I didn't care if the sun came up for me or you. I had no compassion. I knew no limits. I was a dangerous person."

When I met sixty-year-old Jim in 2017, he was a successful businessman willing to generously support the Heart of Dance nonprofit I co-founded to bring partner dance to fifth graders in Duluth, Minnesota. He could do that because he'd spent over three decades building a company that solved industrial-pipe-repair problems, often preventing plant shutdowns and workplace hazards under emergency and stressful conditions.

Jim's generosity was stirred by his love of ballroom dance as "the most fun you can have with your clothes on." His dance teacher described Jim as an elegant dancer with a beautiful frame and as "one of the best dancers in the studio" during his seven years of lessons.

Yes, this was the same Jim who'd been an angry young man. Two things had changed his life.

First, Jim's dad stopped drinking and reunited with Jim's mom when Jim was in his twenties. His father was a mechanical genius. He could fix things and solve the toughest industrial problems. Jim learned from his dad, followed in his footsteps, and become a licensed pipe fitter. At a very young age, he was foreman in a plutonium-recovery plant.

The second thing? A two-thousand-pound buffalo named Nitro.

On Memorial Day weekend of 2013, Jim went with his wife, Jan, and two toddler grandsons to a buffalo ranch south of Duluth to buy meat from his eighty-three-year-old friend, Don. As the animals approached, Jim noticed Nitro, the herd bull, nearby.

"I see you have the big guy here. Are we OK?" Jim asked Don several times.

Don, who had raised the bull, assured Jim that Nitro was simply coming for grain in the barn.

An instant later, the bull charged Jim from behind. The bull gored his left horn inside of Jim's right thigh, exploding the femoral artery. Jim was then launched twenty to thirty feet into the air, clearing the barn roof before he landed.

By some miracle, the bull horn hadn't ripped through Jim's pelvis, and Jim didn't break his neck when he landed. But the situation was still grim. People live an average of two minutes when the femoral artery is hit.

Jan rushed the kids into their car seats and cradled Jim's head in her lap. Don tried to tie off the bleeding, but to no avail.

He looked up. "Honey, I don't think I'm going to make it. Make sure everyone knows I love them."

Then another miracle happened.

Don began to pray, and suddenly he remembered a book he'd read twenty years before about the first heart transplant, performed by Dr. Christiaan Barnard. The book said that they'd lost early transplant patients because "there weren't enough hands to stop the bleeding." So Don thrust his hand inside Jim's wound—elbow deep—to squeeze off the blood flow near the pelvis.

When the county firetruck arrived, they loaded Jim and Don up together. But the ramp and right lane of the highway were coned off for upcoming construction, and holiday traffic was backed up for miles. Thankfully, the road crew opened the ramp and lane for the firetruck and their state trooper escort. It still took an hour and five minutes to get to the hospital. Jim was conscious throughout, with Don at his side, unwilling to let go.

Jim was in the ICU for five days. One shoulder was fractured; the other, dislocated. Both rotator cuffs were torn. Leg nerves were cut.

Though doctors took a vein from Jim's good leg to replace the femoral artery in the bad leg, they predicted they couldn't save Jim's leg. They expected he'd need several months in the hospital. They also expected that he would never walk again.

Jim would have none of it. He walked out of the hospital twelve days later.

It wasn't a good choice to go home, of course. The pain felt like searing fire, without respite. Then the leg swelled so much that it wasn't recognizable, infected by both the bull's horn and Don's hand.

It took surgery, implanted drains, and nine more months for the swelling to subside. And all the while, there was constant pain, twenty-four hours, every day.

"If I let it," Jim added.

Jim's leg was starting to atrophy. He went to physical therapy and Pilates "so the left side of my body could teach the right side what to do." But there was no brain connection to his right leg. And once the nerve stopped feeding the muscle, it would be all over.

Jim knew he needed something more. How could he keep the muscle alive?

He bought a cattle prod.

"I whacked every trigger point from my hips to my toes three or four times a day with an electric nine-volt hit to keep the muscle alive," he said.

That seemed to work.

When Jim's physical therapist was summoned for lengthy jury duty, Jim began working with another therapist. This new therapist suggested he meet dance instructor Andrea Kuzel, who had recently opened Superior Ballroom Dance Studio in Duluth.

On January 5, 2014, Jim hid his walker in the car, propped himself up on the wall, and walked into the studio while downplaying how badly he was hurt.

"I told Andrea I needed to learn to reuse my leg," he said. "We started with a waltz box, and I stepped forward. 'Take a sidestep,' she said. I couldn't. There was no brain connection in my right leg. She reached down, grabbed my leg, and it took a step. I then moved my left leg. 'Take another step,' she said. I couldn't. While holding me up, Andrea moved my right leg backward. We did this over and over. It took me three weeks to master a waltz box step."

Jim spent hours practicing his waltz box in front of the studio mirror, sometimes ten hours a day. He thought if he could watch the movement in the mirror, he could grow a new set of nerves in his brain cortex to connect with his leg.

Jim was in the fight of his life. "Andrea was my angel. She has a genuine care for people that not many people have. What she created for me was a safe place to learn to move and walk. I was taking that pain to a safe place—and taking myself out of my engineering stuff and my practical mind, where I'm the guy who figures out everything. Had I stayed there, I wouldn't have been able to heal. I got on this whole other track with dance that I never experienced before—the creative side of my brain."

It was all new for Jim. He'd never before listened to music. He'd never opened up to people he didn't know well. In his line of work, he doesn't talk with people. He fixes gas, acid, and other leaks—stuff that people don't want to go near. No one questions him. He's the boss. He doesn't have to discuss things with people.

"I never went to high school," he added. "Dance was the first school I went to. Now young girls are scolding me, and I'm cracking up because *no one* scolds me. It was hilarious. This is like finishing school for me. I come in all rough, and they're teaching me how to talk to women. Dance removed me from myself and took me into this big dance ball. Wow—so good for the spirit. It completely encompasses you, and you can't escape it. This was as much of the healing as anything else."

As for Andrea, dance is about making lives better. She had no idea she was doing that at first—in part because she didn't fully understand the impact of Jim's injury.

"Jim told me, 'I got attacked by a buffalo,'" she recalled. "He showed me where he lost a hand-size chunk of tissue. He talked about managing pain. I would feel his leg, and it was on fire. He said it was like having a curling iron on his leg. Yet he was always so matter-of-fact! There were some days when he just needed to dance, and I realized he must be having a bad pain day."

Jim continued to dance—Smooth and Rhythm, solos, whatever. He even won "Top Newcomer Male" at the Snow Ball dance competition.

"Our whole time together was seven years," Andrea recalled. "He's so fun to dance with. He's a great student. He listens. There's no ego when it comes to dancing. Ego goes out the door. Jim was one of the only students I've had who didn't hear music when he started. He didn't hear the beat! But he trained himself, listening in the car. He was physically fit and strong, so he could hold an elegant frame. He used dance technique to train his muscles, and he knew he had to train them properly."

❧

Today, Jim is back to running his successful business with his son. He developed a whole new company during the pandemic.

Though now refocused on his business, he will always hold a special place in his heart for dance.

"I'm a dancer," he said. "It got me to where I needed to get. I have this wonderful thing for the rest of my life."

And how is he doing physically?

"I have a lot of muscle tone in this leg now," he said. "I believe my main nervous system has integrated. I'm healed. My nerve and shoulder pains are down to almost nothing. It was an absolute miracle. I'm the last person I would have chosen for miracles. Miracles are flying around so hard and fast, we don't even see them because we're all closed up and busy. I think it's because I'm willing to open up and let miracles happen. There is a loving God out there."

Andrea believes there was more to account for Jim's remarkable recovery than just divine assistance. Jim, she claimed, took his healing into his own hands, as the super problem-solver he is.

"Jim never has a bad attitude," she explained. "If *any*one asks him how he's doing, he responds 'Better than I deserve.' He has a heart of gold. He never placed blame anywhere. To not hold resentment toward the farmer who assured him the bull would be fine is a different level of forgiveness. To me, that's amazing. That's Jim. He's an amazing guy."

Yes, miracles are flying all around Jim. It seems he created a few of them himself.

Chapter 6

⌄

The Climb

I settled in to watch my friends Dr. Paul Cederberg and his teacher, Meghan Afonkin, dance their showcase routine at a local dance event. Paul, an orthopedic surgeon for over thirty-five years, was the consummate gentleman. It was a pleasure to dance and socialize with him and his wife, Mary, at events.

Perhaps this familiarity was why I was unprepared for what I saw.

Paul started dancing in the middle of the dance floor to the song "The Climb," originally by Miley Cyrus, while Meghan remained in the audience. This version was sung by Joe McElderry, winner of the British show *The X Factor*. Paul's lyrical waltz-like movements—all by himself—showed strong control, balance, and technique at a mid-to-advanced level. He danced solo *for a full forty-five seconds*—rare in the ballroom world.

Then he paused for two musical phrases so he could reach down, lift his right pant leg above his knee, and secure it to the Velcro he'd personally sewn into the pant leg above.

Paul revealed a prosthesis. We saw a leg with no fibula and virtually no calf. It was two inches shorter than his left leg.

I'd had no idea. Nor had many in the audience, who audibly gasped.

Meghan then danced out to join Paul, and they launched into the most moving lyrical routine I've seen. Tears came to my eyes. Paul and Meghan were so elegant, so smooth. Not a hint of any obstacle.

The lyrics of the song made me imagine the uphill battle of climbing up a grand mountain. It was all about the climb—not so much about what was on the other side.

And of course Paul had chosen this version of the song, sung by a male. This was Paul's story. Not just his dance story but his life story.

"'The Climb' is a metaphor for overcoming obstructions," Paul said. "Overcoming whatever is in your way or bothers you. Because we all have those problems. It's the theme of my life and everyone's life. Literally, I'm living the dream. I'm doing everything I've taken on as well as possible with God's grace."

Paul felt that theme hit him hard during the dance routine.

"The last thirty seconds or so that I'm dancing with Meghan, I'm losing it," Paul acknowledged. "I have to keep fighting not to cry. Afterward I cry like a baby."

I asked Paul how hard it'd been to decide to do the routine. A long pause ensued as he struggled to keep his composure. His eyes were teary as he took a deep breath.

"It was a scary decision. I'm still emotional about it. It was more emotionally hard than physically hard. When I make up my mind to do something, I do it. That's something I've learned by having a so-called disability—which is not a disability. It was emotionally hard to expose myself in front of all these people. My dream is to be normal."

He paused again.

"I'm getting close," he said softly. "My whole goal was to inspire other people. To tell a story. It was something I could do to show a disability but also show how it could be overcome with Meghan's help and help of other coaches."

Those other coaches were Bree Watson, Paul's "doctor of dance"; Nathan Daniels; and celebrity dancer Tony Meredith, who cried the first time he saw the routine.

"On my tombstone, I'll say 'I made Tony Meredith cry'!" Paul said, laughing.

The emotion in Paul runs deep. He was born with a developmental birth defect. He has no fibula, only four toes, and is missing other bones in his foot. He has a tiny bit of motion in his ankle. He does have sensation in his foot, which allows him to feel where the foot is in space. He depends on his knee to feel where the foot is. When he was born, doctors predicted that his leg would be five inches shorter than the other when he stopped growing, at age sixteen.

"Dr. Harry Hall was my hero," Paul said. "He decided we could do something without amputating the foot, to my mother's great relief. He did several operations on my foot to get it into this position. When I was twelve, they arrested the growth in my left femur. There's still a two-inch difference that was left so I could be fit with a prosthesis."

That prosthesis is constantly updated. Currently, the materials in his prosthesis foot are made from helicopter rotors, which means they can bend and deform but then go back to normal.

"I'm the only dancer with two right feet, and I dance on helicopter parts," Paul quipped. One might assume it's challenging to dance with a prosthesis, but Paul says he doesn't even think about it.

"I just adapted to it," he said. "The other day, I was doing a hairpin turn, and my brace broke. It's usually dependable. It's just something I'm used to."

All these years, Dr. Hall has lived large in Paul's life. "Dr. Hall helped me," Paul said. He then paused to control his emotions. "I'm lying in bed at age five, recovering from the operation. Dr. Hall says, 'OK, Paul, wiggle your toes.' 'I can do this, Dr. Hall!' I did what Dr. Hall asked. At that moment, at age five, I decided to be an orthopedic surgeon."

Paul never swayed from his ambition.

"That helped me to be disciplined and focused toward my goal. My parents sent me to a private school, where I could participate in sports and academics. I was captain of my football, hockey, and baseball teams. I played quarterback in football. I was a good skater. And an all-conference pitcher. It was perseverance. I just wanted to do what everybody else does. I always tell my dance instructors, 'I want you to teach me to dance as well as I can.' That's the theme of my whole life—doing things as well as I can."

Paul inspired his dance coaches, including Meghan.

"When I first met Paul, he shared about his leg," Meghan said. "As a teacher who's never experienced something like this, it's scary at first. How am I going to be the best for Paul? But our partnership was quite natural as it developed. What I found is that I didn't have to teach Paul any differently. He amazed me from day one. I would give him everything I knew, and he would try it. Sometimes it didn't work, and we'd have to adjust it. But he never questioned anything. He always said, 'Give me more.' He just wanted to be the best possible dancer he could be. I told him I was in it all the way. I won't hold back because I don't need to."

The dance routine to "The Climb" was emotional for Meghan as well.

"What was most moving for me was the choreography with Paul being out there by himself—not with me holding him, not with me there. I could see it in him, even when we practiced, how emotional this was for him. It was a huge triumph. For me also to stand on the sideline and watch him before I appeared on the floor—I'll never forget those moments. I feel so grateful to have had that experience as a teacher. Every teacher should experience something like that because we take so much for granted being professional dancers."

Paul and Meghan worked on "The Climb" for a year. They were invited to perform it one last time at the most prestigious ballroom dance competition in the nation: the Ohio Star Ball. So in November 2019, they performed the routine before a sold-out Battelle Grand Ballroom, filled to the balcony. In a room filled with the best of the best dancers, they received a full standing ovation—one of only two standing ovations of the evening.

"We touched people," Paul remembered. "A big strapping marine came up to me and said, 'Can I give you a hug?' 'Really?' I said. 'Well, if you need to!' He told me he's on active duty and fighting the bad guys for us. He said, 'You gave me hope that if something happened to me, there's things that can be done to help me.' And another girl I perceived as being emotionally disturbed gave me a hug. 'Thank you for doing this,' she said."

Once again, Paul's voice filled with emotion.

"I was happy we made a connection. It was so much fun to touch people and have them acknowledge that what you did made a difference. I didn't cry after that one—I was at peace."

For Meghan, performing at the Ohio Star Ball was different. "It was powerful," she said. "I've been going to this event with my professional-dancer parents since I was three years old, watching past champions who are now adjudicators in their prime. To be invited to perform with Paul was a highlight of my dance career. This is what dancing is about. It's about inspiring and touching people's hearts through performance and movement, which is very rare for even top professionals to do. But Paul did it."

Along the way, Paul nominated Meghan for the "Second Chance at Life" award at the Galaxy Dance Festival. The award recognizes teachers who work with students with special needs.

"I nominated Meghan because she dedicated herself to working with me," Paul said. "I wanted to inspire people with physical and nonphysical disabilities. My belief is that everyone has something to work on, to overcome. I'm no different. My disability is just more tangible, more visible. I try to raise up people around me, and this was a wonderful way to accomplish this."

Meghan was deeply touched by the nomination. "I was honored that I made an impact in Paul's life and could be part of his story," she said. "I do it because, yes, I love dancing, but more so because I've seen such a change in people's lives . . . in so many different ways. And my own life."

So what's next for Paul?

"I'm pushing the limit on what I can do," Paul said with clear-cut ambition. "I'm not disabled," he said. "I was born with something wrong physically, but functionally, I'm not disabled. I'm not a victim. It's actually kind of a blessing because I have to be so focused on what I do. I'm driven to overcome the physical and also the psychological parts too. I try to elevate everyone around me, whether it's my patients, my teachers, my spouse, relatives, whoever it is. It's something positive to do. And we all need something positive to have in our life."

All this truly describes Paul, the man I've known for years. He's all about lifting people up with his positive outlook on life.

Thank you, Paul, for continuing "The Climb." You're carrying all of us with you.

Chapter 7

⌄

I Don't Know What
"Like This" Is

Prior to her retirement in 2010, Lisa Davis worked in information technology (IT) for thirty years, mostly as a specialist for an Iowa state agency. It was an intense experience that required constant attention twenty-four hours, seven days a week. Lisa slept with her BlackBerry by her bedside.

"You had to be prepared at the drop of a hat to address whatever virus or malware might affect any computers on your network," she said. "Sometimes I would work twenty-four to forty-eight hours at a stretch, without relief. It was like constantly running a marathon."

In 1986, Lisa accepted an invitation from a female friend to attend a dance studio function in Des Moines. She'd never danced a step before. But soon dancing, especially the Friday night parties, became her one true form of escape from work.

"Once on the floor, you're only thinking about dance," Lisa said. "The music takes you away, and you're thinking about the challenge of the dance, not the problems of work. It's like a little getaway vacation."

And there was another benefit as well.

"When I worked in IT, I developed terrible posture," she said. "I have to work so hard to overcome that habit. With exercise, I've made a tremendous difference in my dance posture."

In 1990, the studio Lisa attended in Des Moines came close to shuttering. But Lisa and nine others stepped in to save it. They paid expenses, took ownership as a corporation with a board of directors, and managed operations—everything from hiring instructors to cleaning the studio. Lisa personally took over music recordings and hosting Friday night parties.

Lisa gets it done. She has led a remarkable life both on and off the dance floor. I can personally resonate with her desire to escape work stress and straighten those rounded shoulders. Lots of people start dancing for the same reasons.

And oh—did I say that Lisa has been blind since 1981?

Lisa lost her vision suddenly and unexpectedly when she was finishing up her doctorate degree in auditory physiology at the University of Iowa. Ironically, she was studying the genetics of hearing loss at the time.

The first time she noticed it, she was studying in the library, and she had a hard time seeing. She assumed there was a problem with the lighting. She drove home that night, not realizing she'd actually lost a lot of vision. The next day, she drove to the hospital clinic where she worked. She needed to run some papers for a woman registering—again, ironically—for the eye clinic. When Lisa stood up and turned around, she bumped right into a pillar.

"I didn't see that pillar," Lisa said. "When you lose your vision, you don't realize it happened. People think it's like seeing dark or black. That's not what it's like. There's nothing there."

Lisa never drove her car again. Today, she has a very narrow field of vision in her left eye. "It's like looking through a soda straw," she described. She has no vision in her right eye.

The underlying cause, Lisa explained, came from being born three months premature and receiving too much oxygen, which caused retinal damage. She was only a pound and a half at birth.

"I knew I had underlying issues, but I never thought it would result in losing vision altogether," she said.

Lisa finished her doctorate coursework but couldn't complete her research with animals for her dissertation. She had to change her career.

As a newly blinded person, she enrolled in nine months of training from the Iowa Department for the Blind. Upon completion, the department hired her for their adult Orientation Center. That's where blind people develop positive attitudes and self-confidence about blindness and learn how to do things without vision. Lisa taught Braille and computer technology, just as computers were brand new on the scene.

The Iowa Department for the Blind had one of the first local IT networks in Iowa, and they needed someone to support it. So Lisa moved from her role at the Orientation Center to a role in IT.

I never imagined that a blind person could have such a successful career in IT. But Lisa did it.

And what about dancing without vision?

"The dance community in Des Moines had a wonderful group of people who could readily relate to me," Lisa said. "If they sense you're OK with your blindness—that it's nothing more than a physical characteristic, like blue eyes or brown hair—they in turn become more comfortable. You learn to ask for assistance easily and simply, and people catch on quickly."

And because their dance group featured more women than men, Lisa also took it upon herself to learn the leader part in the different dances. She even had a woman dance partner for practice and one competition.

"I do a lot of leading at social dances—it's just plain fun," she said.

But how do you *lead* when you're blind?

"I had confidence that I knew the shape of the room," she said. "You can hear when you're getting close to a wall. There's a change in the sound and the feeling of air. I'm not always successful. It's more challenging in competition, with so many people on the floor. Partner signals help."

And what about dancing with instructors? Lisa has been dancing and competing with professional Markus Cannon for fifteen years, ever since she helped recruit him to teach at the Des Moines Ballroom.

"I'm a good follower," Lisa said with a chuckle. "I can feel if a hair on his head moves."

Lisa's unique circumstances have even helped the instructors be more precise with students.

"When an instructor says 'Do it like this,' that doesn't mean anything to me. I don't know what 'like this' is. You want specificity. You ask for instructions. Right foot, pointed toe, forward and diagonal, foot stays on ground, step to side. He can't say 'put your arm here' or 'look in the mirror.' It won't work. The instructor may have to revisit things many times—foot placement, weight distribution, styling—as you focus on new elements. But that's probably similar to how you instruct other students."

It's a challenge that Markus has welcomed.

"Working with Lisa has truly been one of the greatest experiences of my dancing career," he said. "She's an exceptional student who shows traits every professional competitor searches for in a competitive partner. Her knowledge of musicality and her emotional connection to music play a large role in her drive to dance. Lisa has expanded my patience, knowledge, and teaching skill sets because I have to break down what's required of her, using her different figures and shapes. Thankfully, she calls me a 'Master of Metaphors.' I paint clear pictures in colorful ways to illustrate the movements I ask people to perform or the feelings they should develop when correctly dancing a pattern."

Lisa agreed. "He's a Master of Analogy! He provides me with lots of detail, plenty of practice, and, best of all, tons of fun. He's patient . . . oh, so patient!"

Markus noted several "favorite reoccurring moments" he shares with Lisa. "One is when she rests a hand on my shoulder and whispers, 'Mark, this is a Platinum lesson.' That means I opened doors previously closed or foggy, and the bright sunshine of clarity has exposed some phenomenal truth."

Markus also loves it when he sees her grinning ear to ear after he's given her instructions. "She chuckles and says, 'OK, let's give it a try.' That means I just unloaded a school bus full of colorful information when only a shopping cart would have been necessary."

In addition to her vision loss, Lisa has endured other setbacks. In 2000, she was hit by a car while crossing the street to catch a bus.

"I knew I could be run over, or I could jump on the hood. Because of my dancing skills, I had the physical ability and quickness to jump for the hood."

Her agility saved her life, but she was still seriously injured. She flipped through the air over two lanes of traffic and broke the windshield of another car with her face. She lost her right eye, which had allowed limited vision at that time, and a tooth. She eventually needed a hip replacement.

As if that weren't enough of a challenge, Lisa also suffers from Ménière's disease, which attacks her vestibular system and balance. Today, she exercises to restore balance and get her "pieces and parts" back on track. This of course helps with her dancing as well.

"Your body has to be ready to do a technique with enough control and balance," she said. "Markus stresses this. You need to know how your body will react. I'm always trying to do things that enhance my body's ability to be flexible, strong, and to move."

Through all the challenges, Lisa loves the thrill of ballroom competitions.

"I'll never forget my first Snow Ball," she said, referring to Minnesota's national dance competition held the end of January. "It was an amazing event, and I experienced success. Part of it was that I was determined that our studio would have a good showing, so I encouraged lots of people to go. Our studio got a trophy that year, still on display at the Des Moines

Ballroom. It's a special trophy because we were all in it together. I love rooting and cheering for other people. I remember what rooting meant to me in my first competition. To this day, I'll never know who it was rooting for me. It was some studio from Canada, and they didn't know me from Adam. This is what sportsmanship is all about—to root and support people in their perfection, beauty, and performance on the floor."

What does Markus, as an instructor, think about Lisa's challenges on the competition floor?

"I really don't consider Lisa being challenged," Markus opined. "She's fully capable of accomplishing everything and anything she sets her mind to. I sometimes take for granted the extra effort that's required for her."

And what about Lisa—how does she feel about her challenges as a competitive dancer?

"My big fear on the competition dance floor is that I have really long arms, and I'm afraid I'm going to whack somebody!" she confessed. "I feel terrible when that happens. I feel like the Jolly Green Giant."

She has another unique challenge too—her face.

"I did IT work," she said. "I'm used to sitting in front of a computer by myself. I didn't have to smile or interact or show expression to anybody. Have you heard of RBF—resting bitch face? Well, I have one. Some people will practice with their face in a mirror, but I don't have that option. If I'm concentrating a lot, it shows all over my face—and it doesn't look like I'm having a good time."

So many setbacks, yet such positivity. Now in her mid-seventies, Lisa still exercises three to four hours per day and practices dancing at home.

Thank you, Lisa, for rooting for me and so many others on the competition dance floor. Please know that many of us are rooting for you, on and off the dance floor. You inspire us with your perfection and beauty—both inside and out.

Chapter 8

⌄

I Can Stand Straight,
Both Inside and Outside!

We often hear about midlife married couples who find new joy together in ballroom dance once their children leave the nest. But for Regina Kim, ballroom dance was the unexpected remedy that lifted her out of darkness and depression after her children left home and her increasingly abusive twenty-five-year marriage ended.

Ballroom dance was "totally new" to Regina. She'd never even heard about it in her native South Korea. But she started her dance experience at age sixty in Minnesota with an instructor who kept reminding her, "Regina, posture!"

"I realized you have to show off yourself," Regina admitted. "It gave me confidence that I could do this. That was a big joy! It's like my self-esteem was coming back. I can do anything. This is my life. And I can express myself. I can stand straight, both inside and outside. I realized I was the one who can make me stand straight, make me who I am, and make me a happy person."

Dancing allowed Regina to rediscover who she'd been before her marriage, back in Seoul. Young Regina had a great job as a financial professional with a global company. She was poised to rise through the executive ranks. Korean society is male dominated, so it was rare for a woman to have such a position in business.

"I was very proud of myself," Regina said. "Everyone told me I was doing well, and my boss wanted to promote me."

But life sent Regina on a detour that would lead her far from Seoul. It began when Regina connected with a girlfriend from Seattle who traveled to South Korea monthly for her husband's business.

"We were partying and drinking," Regina explained, "and my friend asked if I had a boyfriend. I said no. So I gave her my business card and told her 'I'm willing to meet anyone if the right one is out there.'"

A few months later, Regina received a detailed, five-page handwritten letter in English with photos from Bob (not his real name), a man in Minnesota who worked for a German company.

"I was completely shocked," Regina said. "He even wrote one sentence in Korean. I didn't know who he was."

As it turned out, Regina's friend had met Bob at a Korean bar in Seattle. At the time he was pursuing another Korean woman, but she was married. So Regina's friend told him, "If you'd like to meet a girl from Korea, I know a really good one."

Regina realized that Bob was serious. He wrote well and was well-educated. So she wrote back, in part to practice and improve her English. Letters turned to occasional phone calls, which then turned to nightly calls. It amounted to a long-distance phone bill of about $1,000 per month.

"He was good at speaking," Regina said. "He had a really calm voice. He was really nice. And my English was getting better."

Regina wanted to meet Bob in person. She arranged a trip to Canada to visit her sister, and then Bob sent her a ticket to Minnesota.

"We had a big rendezvous," Regina said. "He took me to his parents' house and showed me around Minneapolis. During that time together, I was like a magnet."

Regina liked the way Bob's father acted toward his wife. He

seemed like "such a loving husband." She thought that boded well for her promising relationship with Bob.

Bob proposed to Regina when she returned to South Korea. She said yes, against advice from her parents and work colleagues, who said she was "crazy" to give up her family and career.

"I told my father, 'Life is a kind of gamble,'" Regina said. "I didn't have anyone I loved at the time, and I really loved this guy. He was from a good family. He was smart, and he could take care of me. I really wanted to start a family, and I always wanted to live somewhere other than Korea because I'm curious and adventurous. I can do anything. I said, 'If I fail, I'll come back and start again.'"

Regina came to Minnesota in June 1991, and she and Bob got married two weeks later. Bob had prepared everything in advance for a wedding at his sister's farmhouse. Regina's only family in attendance was her sister from Canada and her sister's boyfriend.

"That day, I was the happiest woman in the world," Regina recalled, smiling at the memory.

They had two children right away: Trever in 1992 and Allie in 1994. Regina worked for Bob's business. Things were good for seven or eight years.

Then things started to drift apart. It was "like a little crack that grew bigger." Bob began to dominate the marriage. Regina tried to follow his lead, which meant letting go of her own opinions. She became less extroverted and less "brave." Though communication was an issue, she focused on her children.

But the problems became even more evident after the kids left home. Regina was unhappy working with Bob, and she had nowhere to go at the end of the workday.

"It wasn't a happy marriage," Regina said. "He was putting me down in front of people, like the employees and our kids. Everyone knew it wasn't a good marriage anymore. And when we were both out together, I just couldn't take it anymore."

Regina felt demeaned, especially when Bob berated how she spoke English, her second language. She sought counseling.

"The counselor asked me, 'What would you do if your daughter was in a marriage like yours?' I said, 'I would tell her to get out.' The counselor responded, 'If you don't get out, what message are you sending to your daughter and son?'"

Then came March 27, 2015, when Regina crashed her car on a snowy and icy highway. Though she was driving slowly, her car spun out of control. She was seconds away from being smashed by a big pickup truck.

"It was a miracle I wasn't killed," she said.

Shaking from the shock, she called Bob, telling him about the accident and how she thought she was OK. But he responded with an outburst: "Now I have *three* kids!" He was scolding and raging mad. When she asked if he could pick her up, he replied, "I guess so."

"I felt like somebody was telling me there is clearly no love," Regina said.

The couple divorced in October 2016. Regina wasn't working, and she lived in a rented apartment. She felt empty yet "light" at the same time.

"The reason I was depressed was that I'd had the highest self-confidence when I came here," she said. "This wasn't what I'd planned when I came to this country. I lost huge things. I was sad because all my dreams, my happiness, and my confidence about what I could do when I came over here was a closed chapter. Now that stage was closed, and there was a new stage, but there wasn't anything on the new stage. What am I going to do now? How can I start now? I feel light and free, and everything is in my power, but how can I start my life back? I was losing weight and couldn't sleep."

Regina was now sixty years old, with no family in the United States other than her children. So a friend suggested she try something she'd never done before—dance. "It makes you feel pleasant and connects you with people," the friend said. She suggested the dance parties at a local ballroom studio.

Regina went to her first dance dressed in blue jeans and tennis shoes. She knew nothing about dancing. She had no idea what foot the lady started on. Men would try to help, but they wouldn't ask her to dance again.

But Regina didn't give up. She started taking lessons at the studio, learning a variety of dances.

"I was hooked," she said. "I just loved it. It was a totally different world, a totally different life. It was something I'd never done and never thought I would. When I finished a lesson, I thought, 'Wow, I can do this!' Getting encouragement, listening to music, and meeting people helped me get out of the darkness and depression. And it was really good for my body, having the right posture and movement."

Learning to "stand straight" made Regina confident, happier, and healthier both physically and emotionally.

"That's the way I believe God wanted me to live," she said. "It's also how I wanted to live for my lovely kids and not be their burden. I'm me, and I became a happier person."

New doors opened in other parts of her life as well. She found employment as an accountant with a Catholic school in Saint Paul, where she has worked since 2018.

Dance helped the extroverted Regina emerge again. As she sees it, dance is about connecting with people.

"When we dance, there's a physical connection. We both listen to music while coordinating together. That's a huge plus. Dance makes me invincible! I see as benefits all those micro-movements that connect your brain with your heart. Music always brings me joy. With music, you move your body, so that your heart gets warmed up."

Regina learned of a couples' class being organized by a local dance instructor, but she needed a partner. At an unrelated group class, she noticed that Stefan did the bolero, her favorite dance.

"So I said to Stefan, 'Hi, I'm Regina. They're having a couples' class. Are you free Thursday evening?'"

Stefan agreed, and they became dance partners in October 2021. Bolero is his favorite dance too.

Regina then began taking lessons from the class instructor, Scott Anderson. They performed her first showcase dance—a bolero—in February 2022.

Regina doesn't want to participate in dance competitions but rather dance at showcases and on a formation team. She would love to visit senior housing or recreational parks to show others how dance can create happiness in their lives.

"I want to keep dancing as long as my body allows," she said. "As long as I can walk, I'll be dancing. I want to die on the dance floor," she added with a laugh.

Despite the twists and turns her life took, Regina doesn't harbor regrets. If she hadn't come to the United States, she wouldn't have her children, whom she adores. But while she has no regrets, she admits that she struggled with self-doubt for quite a while. She wondered, "What's wrong with me? Is there anything I did wrong? Should I have done something different to save the marriage?" She especially asked herself these questions when she saw others living a seemingly smooth and happy life.

"I've come to understand that everyone's life is different," she said. "I shouldn't compare myself. That's a big way to take my self-esteem down. I don't want to compare my life to others. I am who I am, and I owe it to myself and my kids to be a happy person."

Today, Regina lives with serenity and gratitude.

"I told a friend, 'I'm a millionaire,'" she said. "I have everything. All my body pieces are in their original places; I haven't replaced anything in my body. There are so many people—billionaires—who have health but emotional problems. I can do so many things. I can dance, which I'd never believed would be part of my life. I don't know what I'd be doing now if I didn't dance!"

PART II

What's Holding *You* Back?

Your reasons not to dance are plentiful and genuine. But what is *really* holding you back? Nearly all beginning and returning dancers face deep-rooted fears and faulty assumptions. Fears can hold back dancers of all ages. What happens when you "peel back the onion" and uncover that hidden fear? Does the fear that holds you back from dancing hinder other areas of your life?

Chapter 9

❧

I Can't Dance Because . . .

Now, I know what you're thinking: *That's great for others, but dance is not for me. I don't have the rhythm. And I sure don't have the time!*

If you've never danced or if you stopped dancing long ago, your reasons not to dance are plentiful, and they seem very genuine to you.

I can't dance because . . .

- I'm too old.
- I'm busy parenting a young child.
- I'm overweight.
- I don't have a partner.
- I have an injury or a medical challenge.
- I have a disability.
- I'm depressed, grieving, or not emotionally ready.
- I'm too busy with kids, my job, and my life.
- It's too expensive.
- We don't do that in my culture.
- I'm gay or trans, and ballroom dance is for straight people.

Are you nodding your head? Then this section is for you.

That list represents some of the most common reasons people list when they say they can't dance. But more often than not, those "reasons" are just cover-ups for the *real* reason: deep-rooted fear.

Nearly all beginning or returning dancers face deep-rooted fears. But once they push past those fears, ballroom dance changes their lives in ways they never imagined. They discover new joy, new community, and new support.

Dance is so much more than you may think. It's all about life. It's an opportunity to break through whatever holds you back from dancing—and likely whatever holds you back in other areas of your life as well. It's an invitation to meet or get more comfortable with your vulnerable self.

Welcome to "unreasonable fears," especially for women. When I started taking dance lessons, I was so in my head. I was ashamed or embarrassed every time I made a mistake, didn't perform well, or wasn't perfect.

It didn't help that I never had great self-esteem in the first place. My parents always had enormous expectations for me, and I felt I never could meet them. But it was more than that. Messages in media, movies, and life made it seem that women weren't smart enough or ambitious enough to succeed as well as men. It felt like beauty was all that mattered for women, but most of us didn't measure up.

In my young adult years, I learned that two-thirds of women of my generation didn't have a strong self-esteem. Ironically, it appeared that white women, such as myself, experienced low self-esteem more often than women of color. How I admired women of strong self-esteem!

For me, the most gnawing fear over my lifetime has been what I call "The Unreasonable Fear of Making a Mistake." A mistake would make me look incompetent and unprofessional. What would people think of me?

It appears I wasn't alone in this. I remember learning about a researcher years ago who gave a mechanical puzzle with no solution to a group of women and to a group of men. The researcher let each group struggle with the puzzle for a set time, then the researcher told them they were "the worst group" he'd ever seen and that he couldn't understand how they'd failed to perform the task. The difference in response between the two groups was stark. "I'm sorry" was the most frequent response for women, followed by "I'm not good at this mechanical stuff." The men, however, would have none of it. "You didn't explain the directions right," they retorted.

Why is it so easy for women to internalize a "mistake," whether or not they contribute to it? I once apologized to a chair when I bumped into it.

Various studies during my young adult years explored why some women "rising stars" shot to the top in their professions while others seemed to plateau along the way. Mistakes were key in that difference. But it wasn't about which women made mistakes. It was about how women performed *after* the mistakes. Those who learned from their mistake and then moved on were most successful. Those who struggled to let go of the issue found that their subsequent performance continued to suffer.

Sounds just like me in my dance career. Sometimes I just couldn't get off the plateau.

But I've been trying. I learned long ago that the most successful people learn more from their mistakes than their successes. Some results work better than others. We learn from the journey. That's how life works.

And it's OK to acknowledge that you have strengths in some areas but not in others. Everyone has different gifts, and no one is expected to have them all. Including dancers. You highlight your strengths in your dancing, then find dance teachers and partners with different strengths to help you create that whole elegant picture.

But my unreasonable fear of making a mistake wasn't my only challenge when I entered that first dance studio. I was also facing "The Unreasonable Fear of Taking a Risk."

Heck, I had no problem putting myself out there to run for public office. That risk was just fine. But OMG, what if somebody saw me, a state senator, struggling in this dance studio? What if these lessons were a waste of money, when I had so many other financial needs in my life? What if these lessons were a waste of time, when I had so many important responsibilities, both personally and professionally? What if I just didn't have talent as a dancer?

I really could get down on myself.

Risks imply downsides, and research shows that women focus on those downsides, just like I did. I wasn't focused on the upsides, the benefits of dancing—other than my goal of finding a husband. I didn't realize there were so many other benefits: good posture, exercise, joy, community, respite from the intense senate life.

Eventually I got there. I realized that framing risk as a new possibility to further your future or your passion is all upside. That makes risk-taking fun.

If you are going to walk on thin ice, you might as well dance!

I'll concede that women acknowledge these fears more than men. But over the years, a few of my male friends have told me that they experience their own unreasonable fears with ballroom dance. Perhaps these fears are also tied to self-esteem. For males, it's the fear of "rejection" and the fear of not appearing masculine.

So let's go back to where we started. You say you can't dance because . . . you're too busy. You aren't physically fit. You've put on a few pounds. You don't have a partner. You're struggling with grief. You're too old. You're too young.

Really? Or are you just fearful of trying something you've never done before?

The stories in this section may help you answer that question for yourself. So come along, and let's do *The Dance of Resilience*.

Chapter 10

Greta's Crucible

Unreasonable fears were front and center for twenty-six-year-old Greta Anderson of Minneapolis when she decided to take her first ballroom dance lesson. It took years for Greta to build the courage and to find the motivation to step into that studio.

Since high school, Greta had loved popular television dance shows. She wanted to dance "so badly." But she never pulled the trigger. She felt shy and self-conscious, particularly about her size. She thought she was a terrible dancer. She would search online for dance classes and buy Groupons. But then she would bail out.

"I was just too scared and could never make myself go," she said. "I was too self-conscious and uncomfortable with where I was in my life. I was scared, and I let that dictate what I did."

She did attend one group class along the way, but it didn't click with her. The instructor made a comment when dancing with her, something like "You're moving like a full grocery cart."

"I can understand now what he was saying," Greta stated. "It was about connection. But that's not a concept for the first day. It fed into my thoughts that I was a bad dancer."

Then a life crucible occurred that caused Greta to overcome her deeply held fear. Her best friend died weeks before her twenty-third birthday.

"I realized life is too short," Greta said. "You're not guaranteed tomorrow. That was always my excuse: I could put it off. I could do it later. I realized you've got to take advantage of things when you can. So for the umpteenth time, I went onto those websites. I found Mill City Ballroom and bought the ballroom primer lesson online."

It was the summer of 2015. On the appointed day, she arrived at the studio. But then she froze. Greta stood outside the ballroom dance studio for ten minutes. She couldn't bring herself to go in.

"I felt like I was going to be sick—I was so nervous," she said. "Then I thought, 'You know what? You can leave. Nobody knows you are here. They don't know who you are. I don't care about the twenty dollars or whatever it was. They can have it. I don't care. You can leave.'"

Greta turned to leave—but just then, out walked teacher Gordon Bratt from the studio.

"Are you Greta?" he asked.

"Yes," she replied.

From that moment on, Greta somehow navigated through her fears and emotions, returning for lessons week after week. She lost twenty to thirty pounds in the first six months, in part from the increased activity.

"But I think it was also a change in mind-set," Greta said. "I was a happier person. Early on, I couldn't imagine being in such body contact with a person, trying to move around the floor. That seemed mortifying to me because I was so self-conscious about my size."

She continued. "One time in the lesson before me, they were working on another student's posture, and Gordon was fixing something. He put his hand on her stomach and adjusted her. In my head, I would just about die if he did that to me. And then sure enough, in my lesson that day, he put a hand on my stomach and readjusted me, and nothing happened. The world kept spinning, and he didn't go away. I survived. It didn't kill me." Greta laughed. "It was a mental shift."

Let's fast-forward one year later.

At the urging of her instructor, Greta entered the Twin Cities Open (TCO) Dancesport Competition as a newcomer pro-am student. Fiercely battling raw nerves, Greta somehow showcased her new skills in nine different dances.

At the end of the three-day competition, the panel of judges named Greta Anderson the recipient of the prestigious TCO "Potential for Greatness" award. It was a huge surprise and boost to her confidence.

"I was stunned!" said Greta.

⌒⊗⌒

As it turned out, the judges were foresightful. Six years later, at age thirty-two and seventy pounds lighter, Greta attended the 2021 TCO and danced elegantly at the Gold level. It was an amazing progression of proficiency in a short time in the ballroom dance world.

"Dance completely changed my life and me as a person," Greta said. "A complete one hundred and eighty degrees. Six years ago, I was very unhappy. I was very lost in my life. I had no direction. I was working a job that had no room for growth. I don't know how it happened. But I've never loved anything like I love dance. It gave me everything. It gave me a passion. It gave me a community. I met these wonderful people who have become dear friends. It was a community where I felt seen and appreciated, and that was huge. It's been the best decision I've ever made."

Greta's confidence grew in all areas of life. She moved to a new job with lots of room for growth, and today she owns her own business. She married Jonas Culkins in 2023. Their first child, Niles, was born in 2024.

Greta Culkins is now a much different person. "Sometimes I feel sad, looking back at the past, at the girl I was before I started dancing. At the same time, I'm grateful because she got me here. She did buy that ballroom primer. She did go. When Gordon asked if she was Greta, she didn't say no. She didn't run away."

Having the courage to step into that dance studio was just the beginning.

"I feel like my life is different in almost every way. I'm more confident. I'm much more of a fighter now than I was before. I don't feel lost anymore. I took dance, and I started trying. I applied myself to something for maybe the first time in my life. It's been a ripple effect for my whole life. Before, I would accept defeat easily and not try. I kind of floated through. I didn't apply myself to anything. Not anymore!"

These days dancing has been put on pause while Greta focuses on motherhood and family life. Yes, life happens. But dance is unique, in that once a dancer, always a dancer. The passion never really leaves. You can *always* come back to it.

Cindy Snyder did just that, as we'll learn next.

Chapter 11

⌄

Life Happens

For Greta and for many of us, life happens and dancing stops. Some of us wistfully wish we could dance again, but we don't. We have all manner of reasons: kids, spousal issues, intense work, increased weight, lack of body fitness. We have the passion, but we don't act upon it.

Not my friend Cindy Snyder.

I noticed her right away as she competed with teacher Scott Anderson at the Silver (intermediate) level at the 2022 Snow Ball dance competition. Her dancing was elegant and graceful. She seemed to float on the dance floor. Her smile was mesmerizing, and her performance authentic and natural. As a large woman, she didn't have the expected body type of a dancer, nor did she wear glitzy ballroom attire. But that didn't seem to matter. She placed well in her competition heats.

I introduced myself as a fellow student of Scott Anderson. Cindy told me she'd started taking private lessons with Scott just three months prior, in October 2021. Then fifty-six years old, she hadn't danced for over twenty years.

Cindy began dancing at five years old. As a petite youngster and teenager, she took lessons in all styles of tap, jazz, ballet, baton twirling, marching corps, and acrobatics. Her team won the 1980 International Baton Twirling Championship in

Hawaii. She danced through high school, joining a touring company that presented a variety show of song and dance at federal prisons throughout the Midwest. She even trained as a dance teacher with Fred Astaire Dance Studios shortly after graduating from college, and she went on to teach and manage a dance studio with her husband until 2000.

Then life happened. All of it. A sickly child. A divorce that required her to sell the dance studio. A change of profession. A lack of physical fitness from years of doing tax returns at a desk all day.

By the time Cindy returned to dancing, her body was no longer that of a dance teacher in her twenties. Initially, that posed a challenge.

"It's a constant battle, trying to get back into any kind of shape to dance," Cindy said. "And it hits me in the confidence side of things because it's harder for me. You don't feel the same gracefulness or that same sophistication. In some dances, where things are supposed to be sexy or sensual, you just don't feel that at this weight. I'm just not at the level of fitness that I'm used to for dance."

But as Cindy kept dancing, she noticed a shift. She lost weight, focused more on her eating habits, and improved her endurance.

"When I came back to dance ten months ago, I was twenty pounds heavier than I am now," she recalled. "I couldn't dance a whole song of anything when we first started doing this. Initially we would do a dance, take a break, do a dance, take a break. Now we can dance the whole time, one after the other. It's taken time, and you just have to keep at it."

The Snow Ball competition was the real test. Cindy signed up to compete in several dance styles, and she thought there would be breaks in between each dance.

"But no!" she said. "We did them in rounds. You did one, two, three, four in a row. Oh my gosh, I could not speak at the end because I didn't have any air! Rhythm—same thing. Even though we were only doing a minute at a time, when you do five in a row, and you've got the adrenaline going, and you've got an audience, you're really sucking wind by the time you get to the end of it. It was really fun, but I had a hard time with it initially. It's much easier now. Much, much easier now. I think it's because of the conditioning."

And what's Cindy's goal now?

"Well, I would love to get back to a good dancing weight," she said. "For me, I need to lose probably another fifty pounds. It's gonna take a couple more years. So I'll just keep dancing every week and stay positive. I think that helps a lot. It helps with less stress in your life. I would love to continue competing forever—until I can't."

Scott Anderson encourages Cindy to keep working at her goals. "It's a pleasure to work with Cindy," he said. "I could see her skill in group class. If I didn't have enough leaders, she was happy to step in and be a leader. She hears the music, and she moves across the floor really nicely, holding her posture and holding her body so she's balanced. She's a good ambassador for the dance community. And she's willing to help beginners. That alone will help her become a better competitive dancer herself. She's giving back to others and helping them, and that's going to make her stronger as well."

What would Cindy tell others who want to reignite their passion for dance after years away?

"Anybody can do it," she said. "The nice thing about ballroom dancing is that you can come to it at any level and improve from any level. So just dance!"

And what would she tell people who don't think they have a dancer's body?

"It doesn't matter," Cindy said. "It doesn't matter because you're not out there necessarily to put on a show. You're dancing for you. Look at the inventor of the Peabody. They named a dance after him, and he was a very barrel-chested, portly guy. I think *everybody* should dance!"

Cindy wants to dance more, but her job and current family obligations prevent that. "You have to start wherever you are," she said. "It helps me to look at my dancing as a process that I can build on over time. I look at more experienced dancers and I say, 'I want to do that.' Someday I will."

No one doubts that.

Chapter 12

⌄

No Partner? No Problem!

It was 2006, and the administrative and executive commit- tee members of a small-town Catholic hospital were in an uproar. They'd just discovered that the chief of surgery was ballroom dancing with the head surgical nurse on a regular basis. Both were married to other people.

"They went through the ceiling," recalled Dr. John Carlson. "Everyone was upset, figuring that Linda and I could not be dance partners without doing *other things* together. They thought they knew what was happening, but they didn't."

The committee called John into a meeting to explain.

"You folks really feel that men and women cannot be friends and cannot be dance partners in contact with each other with- out having other things in mind?" he asked them. "I play basketball and softball with a bunch of guys. If it were guys, you wouldn't be unhappy about this. You're just unhappy because Linda is a woman and I'm a man and we're touching each other and embracing in a dancing sort of way."

John then told the committee in no uncertain terms that this was the way it would be—he and Linda wouldn't stop dancing, and he wouldn't tolerate any more accusations.

"We've done nothing wrong," he said.

The committee finally relented. They even gave John and Linda permission to practice in the hospital, using an empty room that wasn't being used for other purposes.

The truth was that both John and Linda were in delightful marriages. In fact, the two couples were social friends.

John and his wife, Mary Jo, had been married for over fifty years. They used to dance in a community class, loving it until John broke his leg in 1981.

Dancing went dormant for them until around 2005, when they were invited to the wedding of the son of Linda and her husband, Scott. The two couples decided to take swing lessons so they could dance at the wedding.

"We quickly figured out that of the four of us, Scott didn't want to be practicing dance because it was like work," said John. "And Mary Jo couldn't practice much because she had bad knees and a bad back. It was too painful for her. Linda and I found that we both wanted to practice and dance well—to dance technically correctly, which goes with our type A personalities when you're in surgery. There's a right way to do it, and you want to be doing it the right way all the time."

John and Linda continued to take lessons, and they practiced a few times a week. They didn't dance socially, focusing instead on improving their dance technique.

"We pushed real hard to get the full Silver syllabus under our belts and to use a full syllabus in our dances," said John. "So that's where I was and still am."

❧

While John and Linda practiced dance, Maryann Kudalis discovered the dance community. Her husband, Tim, was a Rotarian, so both were involved in Rotary international youth exchanges. When that led to dance activities for the youth, the dancing bug bit Maryann.

In fall of 2010, she started salsa and West Coast Swing lessons at Social Dance Studio. With just one lesson under her belt, she joined a nightclub two-step formation team.

"I was the worst dancer on the team," Maryann said with a laugh. "I was so stressed out that I lost thirty pounds in less than six months. I was dancing constantly, trying to learn nightclub two-step and the routine. I had no clue how to turn. I knew nothing about dancing, absolutely nothing. I was dancing constantly just to get the correct steps to perform. That's what got me going. I got to know people on my team. I ended up with close friends from that team."

Maryann's new friends guided her into the dance world. The men coached her on the dance floor and gave her tips about places she could dance.

Maryann's husband, Tim, wasn't exactly thrilled. Maryann would work all day as a special education teacher, then she'd dance all night. She hardly ate, and she was hardly home.

Tim finally decided to start dancing two years later—"when he got tired of me being gone all the time," Maryann explained. As it turned out, Maryann thought he was a more coordinated dancer than she was.

However, Tim was battling multiple health challenges, including diabetes and heart disease. He had several heart attacks, the first at age thirty. They danced together only about four or five years before Tim became terminally ill.

The dance community became Maryann's safe place to take much-needed breaks from caregiving. They were the people she talked with and cried with as her husband neared the end. A dance friend even connected her to a hospice service.

When Tim passed in January 2017, the dance community physically embraced Maryann with hugs, wrote lovely cards, and came to the memorial service even if they didn't know him.

"It was just incredible," she said as she struggled with tears. "The dance community was huge, really huge, in their support of me."

∿◉◠

John and Maryann first met around 2018, at the weekly group dance classes hosted by instructor Scott Anderson. John usually attended with Linda, but she was having knee problems. She practiced with John occasionally, but it was becoming more and more painful to dance.

Meanwhile, Maryann, now widowed, was attending the classes to have some fun.

"It was hilarious to talk to each of the different men," she recalled. "I loved rotating because they're all so different. Some days, they would crack me up. You end up having a connection with most people in the circle. And with John, I thought we matched pretty well size-wise, as we're both tall. We were dancing together pretty well. I finally asked him if he was interested in practicing with me because I was looking for a practice partner."

Maryann knew firsthand the importance of finding the *right* dance practice partner. Her first dance partner had made her anxious.

"Sometimes I was crying because I wasn't doing what he wanted me to do or because it was my fault that it wasn't going well. That's one reason I felt it was an unhealthy thing. There were a lot of positives about it, too, but I would always have high anxiety. If you have the wrong partner, it's just so unhealthy in so many ways."

Maryann moved on to a second partner, who appeared to be a "quiet, nice man." But as they danced and spent more time together socially, he decided he wanted to be her boyfriend, and he started experiencing psychotic episodes.

"It was so scary when he had an episode," said Maryann.

John, who was around at the group classes, was concerned about her safety. So he was the right partner for Maryann at the right time.

"John was the first dance partner I had who didn't make me cry," she told me.

On John's end, Linda and Mary Jo couldn't have been more supportive.

"John was still practicing with Linda when we first started," said Maryann. "What's funny is that for our first showcase, I was wearing Linda's dress and doing Linda's routines, and Linda came. And Mary Jo was absolutely there. I like her a lot, and she was taking pictures and videos of us. She was so supportive and so lovely."

So there was John with all three women in his life, enjoying dance as participants or audience members.

John and Maryann have now been dancing together over seven years. They dance regularly several hours per week in practice or in group classes, but they agree that family always comes first.

What I find most intriguing about this dance partnership is that John and Maryann are quite different in personality and come to dance from very different perspectives. Yet it works for them.

John is the more experienced and proficient dancer, and he's more detail oriented. While "close enough" is often fine for Maryann, it's not good enough for the surgeon. But as the technician, John appreciates that Maryann is very interested in practicing and learning how to do it correctly, just like he and Linda enjoyed. Teaching seems to come naturally to John. Medical students would follow him in his surgical practice for three months at a time.

"John is way ahead of me," says Maryann. "I'm not as technical or exact as John, by any means. He remembers so well, and he narrates while we dance, especially as I'm learning. I love that most of the time.

"John has so much integrity that I feel safe with him," she said. "I feel everything is very proper. He's a friend, and we can hug because we miss each other. We've gotten to know each other so well. He's the ideal friendship dance partner to me."

For Maryann, dance partnership is simply about friendship and community. Her passion for dance led her to become president of the Minnesota chapter of USA Dance, where she is focused on introducing new people to the dance community. She knows from experience that it's hard—and scary—to set foot in a dance studio for the first time. But she also knows that once you step inside, you discover that it feels familiar.

Everybody is friendly, and you can dance with a variety of people. It's especially welcoming for people who are widowed or divorced, like her.

"It's cheaper than a date," she said. "And you aren't stuck with someone for an hour over dinner or coffee. You don't have to figure out ways to leave when you aren't comfortable. It's just thirty seconds. Rotate, rotate, rotate. It's a safe environment for single people. You can go alone, and it's OK, especially for older women."

As individuals, John and Maryann have each experienced great health benefits from their love of dance.

Before dance, John played basketball and softball for years. This led to painful knees with a meniscus tear and soft cartilage. He had to stop downhill skiing, and knee replacements appeared inevitable.

But then he started ballroom dancing. At first, he couldn't dance a tango. It was too uncomfortable to put weight on a bent knee for that low, lateral motion. But he kept at it.

"With regular ballroom dancing and hard practice, the strength around your knee gets much, much stronger," John said. "The stability of the knee depends on the muscle strength around it, not just the ligaments that hold the knee."

John found that with frequent dancing and practicing, his knee pain disappeared. He hasn't had knee problems since. Now in his mid-seventies and retired from medical practice, he goes downhill skiing five to six days a week at a nearby ski resort.

Knee replacements? Not for John.

Maryann, just a year younger than John, has seen the physical benefits of dance in addition to the emotional support she received as she grieved. She's now more physically fit, her balance has improved, and she stands up straight.

"You walk like a dancer!" John told her.

Maryann added, "My muscles are more defined now than when I was young. In my twenties, I was tall and skinny. Now I'm strong. My back used to feel like it would go out on me every year, but I don't have problems with my back anymore.

The more I dance, the more physically fit I am, and the more willing I am to lift heavy boxes, garden, and shovel."

For John, dance is a technical sport. For Maryann, it's a community. For both, it's about kindness and support. And positivity.

That's good advice for any partnership, whether you're dance partners or life partners.

Chapter 13

―――⌄―――

Dancing Through Grief

We all experience grief in different ways. Depression, loneliness, and inactivity are the norm. But rarely if ever does dance even enter our mind during that difficult and fragile time.

Maybe it should.

Dance is a healer. It heals your body, your mind, and your emotions. You find community and new partnership. *If* you are willing, that is.

Here are three stories that illustrate in vivid detail how dance can reshape your life and mind-set, should you have the resilience to choose to dance through your grief. Or not, if you choose to stop dancing, as I did.

⌒⊘⌒

I was first introduced to Dan Browning around 2015, when he was a reporter for the *Star Tribune* newspaper, based in Minneapolis. His colleague was interviewing me for a story about Heart of Dance, the nonprofit I'd recently cofounded to bring the benefits of ballroom dance to fifth and eighth graders in the schools. (More on dancing kiddos in Chapter 16). During the interview, I learned that Dan had just taken up ballroom dancing and that he was quite passionate about it.

It makes me smile that nearly a decade later, I find myself dancing weekly with Dan in group classes at our mutual dance studio. I know him as a well-trained, elegant dancer who succeeds in competitive dancing.

But I didn't know Dan's heartfelt and inspiring story until I read it in the *Star Tribune Magazine* on June 22, 2021. Here's how the veteran journalist told it:

When I discovered ballroom dancing, it literally may have saved my life. I arrived on the dance floor in 2015 at the ripening age of 59. I was fat and had only quit drinking a month earlier. I had spent several years caring for my wife, who died of a rare and bizarre brain disorder, and the stress had left me in bad shape. The two of us had always talked about taking dance lessons but we never got around to it. Seven months after her death, I went to hear some music with a woman from my caregivers' support group. She asked me to dance, and I had to confront the fact that I didn't know how. I decided it was time to learn.

I wandered into Cinema Ballroom in St. Paul intending to learn a few social dances, but the first lesson left my head spinning. When the instructor explained the cost of various packages, it didn't register. All I could say was, "Where do I sign?"

Within a few months, I was taking weekly private lessons and as many group classes as I could swing. I danced two or more hours a day six to seven days a week. I shed more than 30 pounds. I eventually faced the terror of asking strangers to dance at the ballroom's dance parties. And when my instructor asked me to perform with her in a recital known as a "showcase," I quit my lifelong martial arts studies. I figured it was the only way I could learn the six dances she had in mind. One year later, I entered the Twin Cities Open, the first of my many DanceSport competitions. . . .

My first personal experience with dance, in junior high gym class, left me feeling inadequate. And I am. But it turns out, so is everyone else. A dancer's grace is achieved through hard work and sacrifice. And yet, it produces a high that few other activities match. . . .

I mentioned that dancing may have saved my life. After decades of martial arts training, my joints were wearing out. I had a rotator cuff tear (which I just repaired), no ACL or medial meniscus in my right knee, and arthritis in both wrists. Not long after I started dancing, I suffered a series of kidney stones, bouts of vertigo that nearly sent me through a wall, and a [stroke]. Through it all, I kept dancing. I decided if death was coming, I would rather go out on the dance floor. . . .

I regret deeply that I never got around to dance lessons with my wife. After she died, I vowed that when someone asks me to do something new, if I didn't have a good reason to say no, I would say yes. Now I'm asking you: Would you like to dance?

As Dan tells it, dancing provided him both a new life and a second career. He began photographing dancers, which rekindled a lifelong interest. He then started Danzante Photography, a dance photography company.

Dance has carried Dan through the grieving process to several new chapters in his life, including a new life partner. And like Melinda and Roger Martin in Chapter 4, Dan discovered that his passion for dance has created a purpose for him. It keeps him dancing "until the end."

Yes, I've heard many a dancer tell me, "I'd rather go out on the dance floor."

You can count me in that group too.

～◎～

As I grow older, I find it's important to let my mentors and others know how much they've influenced my life. So when I traveled to Washington, DC, in June 2022, I made a point to look up my political mentor, Mike Berman, and invite him to lunch.

That's when I discovered a totally unexpected—and moving—story of dance and grief.

Years ago, Mike opened the door to my political career, though he didn't know it. He hired me for my first summer political job as a secretary for the 1974 reelection campaign of Minnesota governor Wendell Anderson.

I remember being in the middle of everything and absorbing everything I could, like a sponge. Mike encouraged me to take on new challenges and to volunteer for some campaign advancement duties. I loved it.

I went off to Duke Law School at the end of August. After my first year in law school, the governor's office hired me back to work on various issues for the summer. I was well on my way to a political career. I remain grateful to this day for the support and interest that Mike took in me, a young woman.

When Walter Mondale became vice president to President Jimmy Carter, Mike moved to Washington, DC, to become the vice president's legal counsel and deputy chief of staff. Following that, Mike continued his deep involvement in politics with the Democratic National Committee, and he founded the Duberstein Group, a highly respected government affairs consulting firm. He's also the author of the well-read online newsletter *Mike's Washington Watch* (www.mikeberman.com) and the book *Living Large: A Big Man's Ideas on Weight, Success, and Acceptance.*

When we met for lunch after so many years, Mike had lost considerable weight. I knew that his beloved wife, Carol, had died in 2007. But I had no idea that Mike was also a dancer. Such a small world.

Here's Mike's loving memorial to Carol on his *Washington Watch* website, written one year after her death:

On August 3, 1964, Carol Podhoretz and I met and had our first date. It was a blind date engineered by my sister, Sheila. When Carol first cast an eye on me, through the peephole in her apartment door, she decided that she was ill and could not go out.

The fact that she was dressed to the 9s let me know instantly what had happened. She had assumed I would look like my sister, who was pretty and slim. Instead she saw a not all that tall, bald man, who weighed nearly 300 pounds. This had happened before and was why I avoided blind dates. But Sheila had been persuasive. Carol was teaching a speech pathology practicum course in which Sheila was a student, and Sheila said it would help her if I took out this new woman in town.

Rather than be totally ungracious, Carol invited me in for a drink, and after an hour of conversation said she was feeling better if I still wanted to go out. We went out for an evening of dinner and dancing.

From that night on neither of us dated any other person and on December 19 of that year, Carol proposed and I accepted. On Christmas day, her birthday, I presented her with a ring. Just over a year after we first met, we were married. . . .

I miss our dancing. Carol had done a stint as an Arthur Murray instructor and my folks had taught me to be a respectable ballroom dancer.

We danced on our first date. We were dancing on December 19 when Carol proposed. We danced in our living room when no one was around. We danced at dances and parties. We danced out-of-doors. We could dance with or without music; we so knew each other's moves and rhythms.

Wow.

On January 12, 2024, just a year and a half after our lunch, Mike Berman passed away at age eighty-four. When I heard the news, my emotional heart swelled with gratitude that we'd had that chance to reunite in 2022. Mike is survived by his second wife, Debbie Cowan, whom he married in 2012. They, too, had danced throughout their years together.

Thank you, Mike, for your profound impact on my life. It continues to this day. By sharing your dance story, you will continue to inspire others.

❧

I have my own story about dancing through grief—or *not* dancing through it, actually.

I stopped dancing around 1998, when I ran statewide for Minnesota attorney general. I lost in the Democratic primary election. I still wonder why I didn't go back to dance after that election. In fact, I didn't go back for *fourteen more years.* Through that time, I did find respite by performing in community theater, but not in ballroom dance.

Upon reflection, I wish I had. My own cumulative grief journey was already beginning in 1998, and it would last through 2003. During that journey, no fewer than five close family or friends passed away.

One of my best friends and bridesmaids, nature photographer Nadine Blacklock, was killed in a car crash during my 1998 attorney general campaign.

My brother-in-law jumped to his death from a hospital window in 1999.

My mother passed in May 2001, and my father in September 2001, just five days after 9/11.

And my favorite cousin, with whom I'd lived growing up, passed two years later.

Of course, I assumed I needed to be that strong woman who was always the problem solver and never needed help. But grief is cumulative. And if you don't deal with it, it comes out in other ways.

I would explode at the most minuscule things. One time, I berated a vendor for not having the right frosting design on the cookies I'd ordered for a nonprofit event.

Most seriously, I broke out with an all-body rash that landed me in the hospital in October 2001. It itched like crazy, and I needed intravenous treatment for several days. When my husband visited me at the hospital on our wedding anniversary, I was wrapped from head to toe in what looked like a space suit. Pretty romantic!

The medical team suspected the rash was in part psychosomatic, resulting from stress. Grief counseling helped me get back to earth. And for the first time, at age forty-eight, I began working out regularly.

But I didn't go back to dance.

Again, I wish I had. Especially now that I've heard these stories of dancing through grief from Dan, Mike, and others for this book. If only I'd known. I'm sure that dance would have been a huge stress reliever at that most difficult time in my life.

And dance would have given me much-needed community—a community of dance partners and dance allies. That's different than dancing solo like in line-dancing or even ballet.

My ballroom dance friend Alicia Keyes recently opened my eyes to this distinction. "With a dance partner there is a true opening of yourself—that's where true joy comes from. It's about touching another person, inviting them into your very personal space," she said. "It is a gift. You are giving yourself to another person to try something together. Being that vulnerable is your gift to that other person and you also receive their gift of vulnerability.

"This level of communication is something we can't experience anywhere else, yet we do it here when we dance," Alicia continued. "I dance to be able to connect people with my authentic self. What I receive back is kindness. The community part is also where we care about each other. That happens because we are vulnerable with each other, which you must be to put yourself into someone's arms.

"That's the invitation of partner dance. The invitation to dance and be vulnerable. I invite you to be vulnerable with me," said Alicia.

How elegant. She's right. An invitation to be vulnerable. And boy, was I vulnerable then. And an invitation to be authentic. I needed that too. But I just didn't know.

Why did it take me so long to go back? It's still a puzzle. I'll reflect more upon it in Chapter 19.

Chapter 14

Channeling Grief Through Dance and Action

There are those who channel their grief into movement on the dance floor, and then there are those who channel their grief into action well beyond the dance floor. One of the most moving experiences I've had in the dance world was working with the Westlake family to create something good—a lasting legacy—out of a tragic loss.

They were three brothers from Rapid City, South Dakota. Fiercely competitive. Fiercely loyal. Driven by rules. Pulling—and sometimes pushing—each other to their personal goals.

By their early twenties, all three were rising to the top of their shared sport of ballroom dancing. Yes, ballroom dance. And not just any style but the most formal, most technical, most rules-driven style there is: International Ballroom dance.

Imagine three brothers competing together, dressed in formal black coattails that frame their partners' elegant ball gowns and dance wings. Any one of the three dance duos could come out on top.

Three brothers, eight years apart. Pete, the eldest—always the leader, always the organizer. Nic, the second—full of energy, a people connector, always talking of going into politics some-day. Seth, the youngest—always happy, laughing at anything, the all-out sports guy who started soccer at age six and ran track and cross-country.

Competitive? You bet. All of them. It's easy to compete with your favorite people. You want them to be the best, so when you beat them, you beat the best. That way, you're just a little bit better than the best. (*He* can be second place. *I'll* be first.)

But as competitive as they were, they were always consid-erate of one another and others. Always opening doors to the ballroom dance world for hundreds of friends as early as their high school years.

Pete and Nic started dancing in high school because they wanted to attend their all-school prom. Upon graduation, Pete enrolled in the University of Minnesota (UMN) and quickly landed in its ballroom dance club, leading it as president for three years.

"I enjoyed organizing and making sure other people could dance," Pete said. "We did a lot of good things to get better lessons for everyone."

Through the club, Pete met national ballroom dance champions Nels Petersen and Theresa Kimler, who provided coaching and gifted resources to the university club. As Pete explained, "They certainly made dancing easy for us college students."

Under Pete's leadership, the club membership grew quickly. Soon, the club introduced its first competition team.

Nic took a different route. He chose not to attend college, having picked up computer programming quickly from the internet. During Pete's junior year, Nic decided to move to Minnesota full-time, in part to enjoy dancing.

"Somebody once told me that the only reason Nic wanted to dance was to beat his older brother," Pete recalled. "I think that was probably true. It was good for me too. He made sure I never rested on my laurels. Nic was right there, nipping at my heels. If I sat around too much, he would beat me. Yes, he did beat me a few times in our amateur days after college."

Seth, meanwhile, was pretty scared of dancing, being six years younger than Nic. But he would brag to others about his dancing brothers. At age sixteen, Seth visited his brothers in Minnesota, and they gave him a dance lesson. It was his first introduction to ballroom dance.

In turn, Seth came to Minnesota to enroll at the university. He was excited to spend more time with Nic, whom he hadn't gotten to know well growing up.

"I bet I can get you to try the ballroom dance thing," Nic told Seth.

Nic gave Seth free lessons so he could partner with a friend at a competition. Seth loved it. He worked with Nic most weekends, then auditioned for the UMN Ballroom Dance Club team. By that time, the club had grown in size and quality, thanks to the strong foundation of Pete's prior leadership.

Just how unlikely is it that three brothers could make their individual marks in the competitive dance world? Very. Clearly, they all shared talent, discipline, and thought process. All three had danced their way into the highest echelons of ballroom dance.

It's not a coincidence, too, that all three pursued careers in information technology. Technology is all about rules, structure, and detailed perfection, just like International Ballroom dance techniques.

Pete continued his dancing in New York and married his UMN Ballroom Dance Club partner, Sehyun Oh, in 2017. Meanwhile, Nic and his partner and fiancée, Neli Petkova, moved up to seventh in world International Ballroom rankings.

Like Nic, Seth remained in Minnesota with his dance partner. He had a dream—he looked forward to the day when all three brothers would compete on the same dance floor of a national ballroom dance competition.

Who knows which brother would have won Seth's dream competition?

But sadly, Seth's dream was never realized. On July 15, 2017, tragedy struck.

Nic, Neli, Seth, and other dance friends finished up a dinner meeting hosted by coach Nels Petersen. Seth went his direction, and Nic and Neli went theirs.

What happened next was caught on video, and the evidence was clear: The driver of a light-rail train ran a red light at a busy Saint Paul intersection and plowed into the driver's side of Nic's car. Nic and Neli were rushed to the hospital.

Seth got the call. Nels and the hospital chaplain met him at the hospital. Neli was severely injured but would recover. Nic would not.

"I had to confront the surgeons," recalled Seth. "There was no signal coming from Nic's brain to prove consciousness. They tried experimental techniques, but no reaction. I felt very cold all of a sudden."

Pete was in Ohio when he got the call that Nic was in the hospital, hanging on only via life support. Pete had unknowingly seen Nic, alive and well, for the last time when he and Sehyun married in New York just weeks before.

"I got up early the next morning and took the longest car ride of my life back to Minneapolis, which is a pretty good haul from Ohio," Pete said. "I fortunately had a little time to be around a piece of Nic even though his mind wasn't the same."

Their parents, Lisa and Bob Westlake, were at a wedding in Missouri when they got the call. They got in the car the next morning.

"They'd been planning to meet Nic and me the next day in Minneapolis," Seth recalled. "They still ended up there, but for the worst reasons."

Together, the family made tough decisions about organ donations and end of life. Sadly, Nic passed two days after the crash. Thankfully, Neli survived, but she suffered severe injuries and trauma.

The light-rail driver was suspended for three days, then returned to his job.

"We were just so frustrated, once we better understood what had happened," recounted Pete. "The driver suffered basically no consequences."

Authorities said the driver's actions did not rise to gross negligence. Investigations confirmed, however, that the driver caused the crash by careless driving and running a red light. So why no consequences for this driver? Because light-rail drivers were *exempt* from the Minnesota traffic code. Had a bus driver run that red light, in comparison, they would have been charged with a misdemeanor.

So began the family's quest to chase legislation at the Minnesota capitol. Changing Minnesota law seemed a natural legacy for Nic.

"Nic was really enthusiastic about politics," Pete said. "He was definitely eyeing opportunities to get into the political world. We also come from a political family."

Their maternal grandfather, Rolland "Rollie" Redlin, was a leader in the North Dakota Senate for over thirty years and served a term in the US Congress.

"I'm sure our grandpa was watching down on us—and maybe he was joined by Nic," Pete added.

The legislative push began in January 2019. It turned out to be a much-needed healing journey for the Westlake family.

"When this legislative opportunity came up, it was, for me, one more adventure with Nic," continued Pete. "It was a chance to have this experience with him—something he would be good at. He would have enjoyed being there with us. If this had happened to any other one of us, Nic would have been shoulder to shoulder with the others, leading the charge to make that change."

"It didn't feel like we were doing it out of anger because we lost Nic, though that was part of the motivation," Seth added. "We didn't want Nic's death to mean nothing. We wanted to cause change that would help other people. It was a good part of the healing, to be able to accomplish something like that in his loss."

The Westlake family created a clear goal and positive message to drive change. But nothing at the legislature is easy.

"Thinking back on it," Pete said, "I was blown away by how hard it can be to get something simple done in the legislature. We put a huge amount of effort into it, to get an obvious thing fixed. It was amazing how much energy that took. On the flip side, I know we had pretty good success, and a huge amount of luck comes with that. We were fortunate that it felt easy."

Easy? The brothers made no less than seven trips to the capitol to testify before committees, watch floor debates, and finally attend the bill signing. Pete flew in for each session from his New York home. Their success came from their dedication and tenacity.

With guidance from Nels, the brothers created a team that believed in them, including lawyer-lobbyist Patrick Hynes and bipartisan bill authors Senator Carla Nelson (R-Rochester) and Representative Cheryl Youakim (D-Saint Louis Park). Nels invited me to join the team during the January Snow Ball dance competition. As a former Minnesota state senator, I was honored to volunteer. I felt I represented the support and love of the entire ballroom dance community.

The legislature can be intimidating for testifiers, especially in senate hearing rooms. As Pete described it, "Most of the time, you're sitting in the middle of a big round firing squad of questioners."

Seth added, "The grandeur of the round table and the senators sitting above you, looking down, was a very different feel from the House."

But the brothers were fearless.

"For me, it was a big adventure," Pete said. "It was something we needed to do, like cracking open a new video game. A new set of challenges to solve problems. We might not be successful, but that never stopped me from playing a video game. You can think of it like dance too. I know that in competitions, I may not be the best. It's great if I am, but that's not going to stop me from getting out on the floor. You can't be afraid to get on the floor."

The brothers' loving bond and fierce commitment were not lost on legislators.

"I'm the mother of three sons myself," Senator Carla Nelson told me. "I'm reminded of scripture: 'A threefold cord is not easily broken.' I often thought that about my sons, and I saw that with the Westlake brothers. They honored Nic every step of the way. After our first hearing, we needed to take a selfie because Nic would always take a selfie. As if Nic was there."

Senator Nelson was deeply moved by Pete and Seth's courage to drive change in the face of their grief.

"What I really appreciated was in their time of grief, they were able to turn that grief into action," she said. "They did so very thoughtfully. Their ballroom dance training prepared them for poise and grace during strenuous times. And tenacity. You want to work with people like that on every bill. They were in such pain, yet they were able to work through that in a positive way. They channeled it for good."

The senate process went smoothly. After two committee hearings, the bill passed the full senate unanimously. That day, Senator Nelson acknowledged the Westlake family, sitting in the senate balcony: the brothers, their parents, and their ninety-two-year-old grandma, wife of the former North Dakota congressman. I was proud to sit at their side, along with Nels and Patrick.

Representative Cheryl Youakim, the House author, also found the brothers to be amazing messengers. But despite their heartfelt committee testimony, the road to bill passage through the House was rocky. Legislative opponents of light-rail persistently tried to broaden the bill with unrelated partisan amendments. Representative Youakim showed extraordinary discipline in keeping to her message and fighting off these amendments.

"This is a narrow bill that the family brought to us to correct a problem that greatly impacted their lives and that will help others," she told her House colleagues. "Let's keep it clean and send it to the governor so the family can have closure."

Amid the chaos, a highly unusual clerical error caused a defeated amendment to be included in Representative Youakim's bill. In order to remove the erroneous amendment, she was forced to debate opponents in the next committee for an hour! That turned out to be the warm-up for a one-hour battle in the House of Representatives, where eight Republican lawmakers rose to support amendments for other purposes.

"I was emotionally frustrated," Representative Youakim recalled. "It should have been a simple fix, but they were playing games with it. That was the first bill I had gotten so personally invested in and emotional."

In the end, all but one House member voted for the bill.

Easy? Welcome to politics.

None of this was lost on the brothers. "Both legislator-authors were amazing to work with," Seth said. "Both were incredible speakers for our case. To see Representative Youakim confront resistance from her fellow House members in a professional and no-nonsense way, that was so good to hear. Sometimes it felt like, 'How can you oppose a change like this?' It felt good to have competent people on our side."

Pete agreed. "We could always tell the authors were fighting for us. I think both adapted to their environments. Cheryl had that vibe of the House. She was scrappier, ready to jump in, bob and weave a bit. You could see more rough-and-tumble in the House. Carla was the picturesque and precise senator. They were perfect fits to present their bills in their environments. It was fun to see them work."

The long road led to a private bill signing with Governor Tim Walz. Unfortunately, only Pete could attend from New York because a winter storm west of Minnesota prevented their parents from traveling from South Dakota. Seth, too, was unable to travel, as he was returning from a dance competition. So the governor dialed up their parents on speaker phone during the signing. Both bill authors and the lieutenant governor attended.

While it was a warm and exciting moment for Pete, it was "strange" to celebrate this big victory lap by himself. He had traveled so much of this road with Seth, their parents—and Nic in spirit.

"I was lonelier than I expected," he said. "Especially the time thinking about Nic."

The group took a selfie, with Pete holding a photo of Nic in a magazine. Framed photos were sent with appreciation to the bill authors.

So how did the brothers manage to channel their pain in such a constructive way?

"We wanted to cause change in memory of not having Nic, so we did have to live through that pain," Seth said. "But this was our way of making meaning out of Nic's death and to honor the brother we lost."

"I honestly felt less sad doing it," Pete said. "I felt so much like Nic was there, especially when we would think about what to say. For me, it wasn't so sad because it was a cool way to spend more time with Nic. It was almost sad to have it over."

In the end, brothers will always be brothers. The legislative journey brought Pete and Seth together in many ways. They recall playing video games at Seth's apartment late into the night after a successful day at the capitol.

"Despite all the important stuff we had to do, we always fit in that time to be brothers," said Seth.

Added Pete, "We had a project to work on, and I could connect with Seth like I connected with Nic on projects. And we could play video games. It was a good excuse to make some time for that."

I suspect Nic and Grandpa Rollie were looking down with great pride—maybe while playing their own video games—and loving it.

Chapter 15

This Is What Keeps Me Alive!

You're never too old to dance. Really. Dance competitions around the country feature the Super Senior level, where seniors seventy-five or older compete.

When dancers say they want to "dance till the end," they *really* mean it.

That's why I was mesmerized when I saw a petite gray-haired woman performing an Argentine tango at a dance showcase at the Mall of America (MOA) in 2021. Though she appeared lighter than ninety pounds, she danced flawlessly, following every kick and every timing change while maintaining picturesque posture. Such a performance would be difficult for anyone, but not for Angela Calabria, *at age ninety-three.*

I needed to meet this woman!

I later visited with Angela at her assisted-living residence in Minnetonka. She explained that she hadn't seen David Salvatierra, her former teacher and MOA dance partner, for three years prior to the showcase. They practiced for just one hour in the hallway before heading to the MOA to perform.

"We practiced a few steps, and I followed him," said Angela. "I said to myself, 'This will be my last hoorah.' I can still dance. People will hear I'm ninety-three and that I have no crutches, no cane—that is unusual at my age. And here *you* are," she said to me, "to hear more."

Angela was right. At my young age of sixty-eight, I was inspired—not only by Angela but by her daughter Alissa Quinn from Albany, New York, who had performed a beautiful showcase of her own at the MOA event.

It all began when Alissa made plans to visit her mother and brother in Minnesota before Thanksgiving. Angela learned it was the same weekend as the MOA exhibition, so she asked Alissa to perform for her there. To make it even more special, Alissa invited her professional dance instructor and also her mother's former Argentine tango dance instructor to join them in Minnesota and provide one last meaningful mother-daughter dance experience.

Both dance teachers responded enthusiastically and rearranged their schedules. The plan took coordination and expense, but everyone was up to the challenge.

"I was very happy it worked out in such a special way," Angela said.

Angela's dance story began approximately sixty-six years earlier, when her sister invited her to a dance studio party in Brooklyn. Her sister was dating a man who was taking lessons there. Angela resisted, but her sister would not hear of it. She knew Angela loved music and dancing; they'd danced at birthday parties when they were growing up in Ecuador. Not to mention, she knew that Angela had taken a few lessons at Arthur Murray Dance Studio.

"What are you waiting for, Angela? Your prince to come?" her sister had challenged.

Well, yes. And her prince did show up.

That's where twenty-seven-year-old Angela met her future husband, Frank Calabria. Frank was one of the studio's ballroom dance escorts for unaccompanied ladies, such as Angela. Angela had no problem following him.

"After a while, Frank stopped dancing with all the other ladies he was supposed to dance with, and I was happy," Angela recalled.

At the time, Frank was focused on writing his thesis to get his doctorate degree in psychology. But every Sunday, he'd pick up Angela to go dancing, have dinner, and see a show. The couple married the next year, in 1956. Shortly thereafter, Frank was hired as a psychology professor for a college in Albany, and the couple settled in nearby Schenectady, raising four children.

Angela and Frank danced ballroom together for over fifty years, learning all styles: Latin, International Ballroom, American Rhythm, and Smooth. Years later, the couple saw an inspiring Argentine tango performance, and they started taking private lessons.

Angela loves Argentine tango. "I love the music," she said. "It's passionate, uplifting, and has the most beautiful music. It's very rich in instrumental tonalities—that just gets my body wanting to dance. The close embrace, that is another thing. I love the close embrace because who doesn't like to be hugged! If you have a good partner, it's the greatest feeling. Argentine tango rhythms can be slow, medium, or quick paced, done three dances at a time, called *tandas*. That gives me the chance to rest in between."

Angela is a woman of spunk, willing to pursue her passion even if it means breaking norms. This happened when Frank underwent a few medical procedures, including back and hip surgeries, that required months of recovery.

"Initially, my husband was reluctant to have me dance with another partner," Angela said. "But if I didn't dance, I was not me. I craved it. I would do it, whether my husband wanted to or not. So one day as he was getting ready for a new procedure, I told him, 'I cannot be happy if I'm not dancing. And just because you're not able to dance, that shouldn't mean I can't dance on my own.' It took me the better part of a year to convince him."

As it turned out, Frank was concerned that she would no longer want to dance with him if she started dancing with a dance teacher.

"I said, 'Just the opposite! If I can dance, I'll be happy, and I'll be happy to continue dancing with you.' The more variety the better! You learn that way."

After a year of trying her best to win Frank over, Angela decided to make the call on her own. "I finally said, 'That's it.' I made an appointment with a dance teacher. And that was that!"

The couple danced at their fiftieth wedding anniversary celebration, though Frank's health was declining.

"We danced an Argentine tango," Angela said. "Frank attempted to do a *gancho*, a hook on my leg, but wasn't able to do it because of my long gown. I have a picture that is so precious, where we're both laughing out loud during our anniversary dance."

Frank passed away in 2010. Two weeks after he passed, a dear friend who was head of the Albany Tango Society called Angela.

"I know how much you love Argentine tango dancing," the friend said. "Would it help if you come and take a lesson with me? A tango instructor from Argentina is coming, and I need a partner."

At first, Angela hesitated. "It had only been two weeks since my husband's passing," she recalled. "I was still in mourning and didn't feel like dancing. But then I remembered that Frank and I had talked about what would happen if one of us passed away. We promised each other that the other one had to continue dancing. So, I remembered that. I said, 'I will.'"

The local and Argentinian instructors came to her home for a lesson. And that drew her back to the dancing circle.

"Frank and I had a wonderful relationship," she said. "He would be happy that I'm still dancing, the way we promised each other."

From then on, Angela focused her dance on the Argentine tango.

Over the years, Angela occasionally visited her son Mark in Minnesota to spend time with his family, including her four grandchildren. When she visited their family in June 2019, she felt a pain in her side as she was preparing to head home. She was rushed to the hospital, where they discovered an acute hernia that needed immediate surgery. She then experienced significant complications, and she ended up in a hospice residence. She believed she was saying farewell to family and friends.

Miraculously, she recovered and was back on the dance floor by the end of the year.

Angela chose to stay in Minnesota, settling in Minnetonka. She discovered the Tango Society of Minnesota, including founder Loisa Donnay.

Since then, as the pandemic has allowed, Angela has attended the Tuesday night milongas at Loisa's studio in South Minneapolis, where she dances with various partners. She also takes weekly lessons from Loisa in the hallway of her assisted-living residence, with Loisa as leader and Angela as follower.

So why does Angela still take lessons at age ninety-three?

"Dancing not only improves my dancing but improves my posture," Angela replied. "And when you laugh, hear dance music, or do things you enjoy, something happens in the chemistry of your body that makes you feel better. I don't feel lonely because I'm looking forward to Tuesday nights or my private dance lessons. Yes, I look forward to my family's visits too. But on a daily basis, dancing is what keeps me alive. I'm not just breathing but enjoying."

And the Tango Society dancers enjoy Angela as well.

"She's a popular dancer because she dances so many things so well," Loisa said. "She can do anything a partner asks. She is very fun to dance with. She is the soul of politeness. She has the manners that we all wish everyone had. She's elegant and dresses so nicely."

How has Angela progressed as a student as her years advance?

"She's sharp as a tack," Loisa said. "She's not as limber as she was in her earlier days, but she's one of the best dancers I have. She catches everything. She's very musical. She's aware of what's going on. She's playful, fun to dance with. It's kind of an amazing thing that the partners just love to dance with her. Her dancing is very responsive to the lead. She can do just about anything. There's hardly anything I'll hold back on. You yourself saw that at MOA," Loisa said to me. "Her instructor did a lift with her—no problem! Just lifted her right up!"

As we'll discuss in Part V, frequent dancing is known to prevent dementia. And Loisa says that Argentine tango is one of the best dances for brain health.

"It's a true lead-and-follow dance," she explained. "That means there aren't as many patterns, as in ballroom dance or a syllabus. It's not a competition-based thing. Argentine tango is a very impromptu, very improvised dance. People feel free to make things up, to create new things. There are so many different things a dancer can do. You have to change your mind all the time, and that's good for you. Getting new input and making a new decision with that new input is what keeps your brain young."

So, what is Angela's advice for older seniors to get them to dance? "I say, 'Why not you? Why don't you start? It's never too late. You can do it. It's never too late to learn something that will give you joy. It's the most complete exercise there is. It uses almost every part of your body, your arms and legs, and your mind. It enhances your posture and your mood.'"

Is dance the secret to Angela's long life?

"Being happy is my secret to longevity," she said. "I have come to the realization that you make your own happiness with whatever your passion is. Your passion can be anything. Mine happens to be Argentine tango!"

～☙～

Angela's long and happy life came to an end on December 23, 2022, when she succumbed to pneumonia at the age of ninety-four. Her obituary recounted her years of dance passion and highlighted her Mall of America showcase appearance, calling her the "Tango Treasure."

I suspect our "Tango Treasure" is happily dancing with Frank and all her heavenly partners as we speak.

Chapter 16

❧

Life Lessons from Fifth Graders

"Out to the cheese. Jump, jump. Back to the crust. Jump, jump. Under the bridge. Jump, jump. Under the bridge. Jump, jump."

This was the chant of fifth-grade dance partners practicing their swing dance steps (on a giant imaginary pizza) during recess at a Saint Paul school in October 2015. And they were good. You should have seen their boogie walks!

Over 250 fifth graders in eleven classrooms across the Twin Cities were completing a ten-week semester of Dancing Classrooms. Dancing Classrooms is a global in-school program that brings the benefits of partner dance to fifth and eighth graders, and this was the first time it was being offered in Minnesota.

With New York–trained Teaching Artists hired by Heart of Dance, a new Minnesota nonprofit, students learned to check their dance positions for "crispy chicken wings" (elbows) and "sticky peanut butter and jelly sandwiches" (touching forearms). The Teaching Artists helped classroom teachers enrich the students' dance experience through essays, poems, artwork, and research into the cultural origins of each dance.

And then the big day came: the first-ever Colors of the Rainbow Team Match in Minnesota. Teams from each school would showcase what they'd learned in a competition before professional ballroom dance judges.

Ten-year-old Emilio, decked out in his classy bow tie and dress pants, was practicing in the on-deck room when he panicked. He was about to dance before a packed ballroom of parents and school teammates. With wide eyes, he ran up to Heart of Dance board chair Dennis Yelkin, the then-seventy-one-year-old gentleman you met in Chapter 3 (who later recovered from multiple myeloma).

"I forgot the tango—show me!" Emilio railed excitedly.

Dennis smiled. "Ask your mother to dance, and I'll show you."

Emilio calmed down quickly as he reviewed the steps with his mother. Satisfied, he ran back toward the ballroom, but then hesitated and turned back to his mother.

"Thank you, Mom!" he said before happily joining his fifth-grade partner.

His mother, visibly moved with tears in her eyes, turned to Dennis. "That is the first time he's ever thanked me for anything." It seems Emilio was learning more than just dance steps.

I'll never forget that day in December 2015. More than one hundred fifth graders on eleven teams jammed into Dancers Studio, creating one of the most ethnically diverse ballroom scenes I've seen in the Twin Cities.

"Their families and friends brought the enthusiasm, shouting and clapping, as if it were an Olympic event," wrote *Star Tribune* reporter Kristin Tillotson.

These young "Olympians" were judged not just on their dance steps but on the newfound confidence, teamwork, and multicultural and gender respect they'd practiced over the past ten weeks in their schools.

Like Emilio, the students and educators of Minnesota had never done this before—and frankly neither had we at Heart of Dance. When cofounder Andrea Mirenda and I sought a license from global Dancing Classrooms to bring partner dance to Minnesota students, we had a dream but not much else.

That didn't matter. The ballroom dance community of Minnesota went all in for Heart of Dance. They believed in our dream. We became the thirtieth global licensee of Dancing Classrooms in July 2015.

As Emilio demonstrated, Dancing Classrooms is all about emulating "Respect, Elegance, and Teamwork" for our youth in schools. How joyful it is to watch these young people break through fear and resistance to "Thank you, partner."

Educators applaud the social and emotional learning components of Dancing Classrooms. As one paraprofessional told us, "Their discipline has gotten much better—not just in dance class. I see it in their other classwork as well. They work better together—more like a team."

Friends and dancers created a founding board of directors so we could get our IRS nonprofit status for Heart of Dance. Multiple donors and volunteers stepped up. Five years later, before the pandemic swooped in, we'd helped transform the lives of 8,706 fifth and eighth graders in the Twin Cities, Duluth, and Rochester at seventy-five partner schools.

During that time, our professional ballroom dance teachers became volunteer "Pro Buddies" and visited our classrooms—often the most memorable experience for students during the ten-week residency. The teachers also served as volunteer judges at our semiannual Colors of the Rainbow Team Match. Like all our donors and volunteers, they believed in our dream of growing young leaders through partner dance.

Leaders like fifth grader Maya, who transformed through Dancing Classrooms from a suspended student in fourth grade to a classroom leader in fifth grade and beyond. Her classroom teacher told us that Dancing Classrooms "did more for Maya in one semester than we could do in three years."

Or like eighth grader Ellie, who found in dance a purpose and joy that helped her overcome her depression and past attempt at self-harm. Ellie became a classroom assistant in a program for alumni of Dancing Classrooms.

Or like fifth grader Harry, a new student at his school. "I was really shy," the youth later told Heart of Dance supporters. "I thought people were going to see my mistakes and laugh at me. But after a couple weeks, Ms. Frances, my dance teacher, made me feel like I belonged there. She made everyone feel like that. I'm not nervous about doing anything now because Ms. Frances made me feel I could do anything. Like, if I want to climb Mount Everest right now, I'll pack my bag, get my food, and start climbing and climbing until I reach the top! I just need to be a little older," he told the laughing audience.

Then there was fifth grader Sam at Windom Spanish Dual Immersion School in Minneapolis. Sam was excited to be selected to dance with his school team in the spring 2017 all-school Colors of the Rainbow Team Match hosted by Heart of Dance. But his friend Luis was really "bummed out" when he didn't make it.

"I thought he should have made it," said Sam. "So I offered to give up my spot for him. I thought 'Well, I'm going to be happy dancing, but I'm also going to be happy seeing him dance. It's like a win-win.'"

So Luis joined the team and came to the elegant ballroom ready to dance for Windom. He then learned that another team, from Learning for Leadership Charter School in Minneapolis, was short a few gentlemen. So he and another Windom teammate volunteered to dance a few dances with the ladies of Learning for Leadership, though they'd never met.

The ballroom was filled with parents and families cheering on the ten Twin Cities schools' fifth-grade teams as they danced the merengue, tango, rumba, waltz, foxtrot, swing, and heel-toe polka. Once again, professional ballroom dance judges judged dancers not only on dance steps but also on their display of "Respect, Elegance, and Teamwork"—the fundamentals of Dancing Classrooms. Once the judges' scores were tallied, every school team received a trophy and every fifth grader a medal.

Luis jumped for joy when Windom placed second in the Team Match. He proudly held the trophy with his teammates, then he texted the news to Sam.

"I thought, 'Wow!'" Sam told a luncheon audience two days later. "Out of ten schools, that's pretty good. I helped them, even though I gave up my spot. Maybe he did better than I would have done."

And then the first-place team was called—Learning for Leadership Charter School! Luis and his Windom teammate were invited to join them for the first-place team photo.

Sam was so proud of Luis. "I found out that my friend was one of two Windom gentlemen to dance with the Orange Team and help them win first place. It was pretty amazing that they did that. I had a bunch of happy feelings all at once."

Add to this story that the first-place team members were 90 percent Somali, and you have a complete picture of how Dancing Classrooms also develops multicultural respect among fifth graders.

Two days later, both teams performed together before more than 220 people at the Dancing with Heart luncheon for Heart of Dance, celebrating two years of Dancing Classrooms.

After sharing his story, Sam concluded, "And now I get to come here and dance with my team after all!"

Yes, the life lessons of Dancing Classrooms are "Respect, Teamwork, and Elegance." But there is so much more.

As Harry said, "If you have a dream and you want to do something, don't stop because you feel someone else is going to think you're bad at it. It just means you probably need to practice. And that's what I did, and that's why I got picked for things."

Harry concluded his comments with this sage advice to his audience: "If you want to do something, don't let anyone else put you down. Just look up and say, 'I'm going to do it.' And when you do it, feel good and give yourself a pat on the back. My mom is here today. She is really supportive. She says, 'Harry, *you're going to make me proud.*' And I tell her, '*Yes I am!*'"

This earned Harry a standing ovation.

Heart of Dance came back, post-pandemic. Students are especially vulnerable after years of disruption. They must continue to dance. And they will. There are so many more young lives to transform—one step at a time.

Chapter 17

❧

Keeping Children Safe

While most children seemed to happily engage in our Heart of Dance classes within a few weeks, we also discovered in our work in the schools how fragile and vulnerable some children can be. For those students who became anxious in dance class due to nonrelated issues in their family lives, teachers and mental health counselors were usually available as resources.

But schools aren't the usual places where young children first learn dance. It is more common for parents to introduce their children at early ages to ballet, tap, or jazz in local dance studios. Parents often enroll their children in dance to help them build self-confidence, poise, and new skills. Parents can drop off the kiddos for an hour or two at a local dance studio, allowing a short respite from parental responsibilities.

Most parents have never seriously danced themselves nor know how to assess the reputation of a chosen dance studio. A dance studio is different from a trusted public school. There are no government regulations ensuring that instructors and other adults are properly vetted and backgrounded. Moreover, the interaction between a child and a dance teacher is more personal and possibly more physical than with a schoolteacher. It's easier to isolate an unsuspecting child in a studio.

All of us have a responsibility to keep children safe from abuse and exploitation. This includes parents as well as the whole dance community. We must lead in ensuring that children have safe and secure opportunities to joyfully express themselves and grow. We can also lead in helping identify the children around us who may be vulnerable to abuse, whether in a home, studio, or any other venue.

That was the key message I learned in a 2022 virtual seminar for dance professionals taught by Alison Feigh, director of the Jacob Wetterling Resource Center (JWRC) of Minnesota, part of the national nonprofit organization Zero Abuse Project. I attended the seminar as the governance and development consultant for both organizations. This chapter is another opportunity to raise awareness. Prevention of child physical and sexual abuse was a passion of mine in my legislative work.

So what is Alison's message? It's a community responsibility to "upstand" rather than "bystand" on behalf of kids.

This message works two ways. Yes, we must do what we can to prevent children from being maltreated or exploited. But we must also do what we can to support those children who have already been maltreated or exploited, including at home.

Dance teachers often don't know whether their students have experienced trauma. Most survivors of abuse do not tell anyone or wait until they're adults to disclose. Rather, the trauma expresses in indirect ways. Sometimes abused youth act out. Sometimes they are overachievers, requesting to stay for extra classes or instruction because the dance studio is a safe place and they don't want to go home.

What can dance professionals, parents, and the dance community do to be trauma-informed? First, we must understand the nature of child physical and sexual abuse. Then each of us can be trained to recognize signs of abuse and what to do about it.

Dynamics of
Child Exploitation

Offenders can be all genders, socioeconomic levels, and cultures, although about 95 percent of sex offenders are male. Most child maltreatment comes from people the child knows. Very few incidents are stranger assaults or abductions, like we hear in the media.

We know some molesters even offend when other adults are present because the conduct is so normalized that the other person doesn't do anything about it. Offenders look for weak spots in studio oversight. They target children who don't get the affection and attention they need at home.

For example, one offender watched how parents interacted with their kids at pickup time. Which kids got loaded into the back seat without a single word of engagement from their parents, and which kids happily told their parents about their lesson as they walked hand-in-hand to the car? It's easy to screen the dynamics around attention or affection.

A single bruise doesn't tell the whole story of possible sexual abuse, criminal neglect, or other abuse, but 80 percent of children who experience abuse in one way often experience it in other ways. People being harmed in person are at greater risk of being harmed online.

Older kids between ages twelve and seventeen are especially vulnerable to sexual harm. At this age, they're becoming more independent, and parents are less involved in their lives. The adolescents look for approval from older adults. During puberty, the brain is still developing. The last part that develops is the part that asks, "Is this a good idea?" A child's gut may say, "Don't give out my address online." But their brain says, "But I get a free game."

This is how grooming works. Offenders skillfully and increasingly break boundaries with the child they're targeting. Groomers look for the weaker child and offer trust and affection, within a seemingly safe social context: "With me you can do this, but only me. You can trust me. I'll keep it secret." Note that once a child is abused by one person, their risk of abuse increases.

The most important way to stop the cycle of abuse is for children to have at least one positive relationship—a stable and committed relationship—with an adult who doesn't abuse them. The adult becomes a place where the child can feel safe.

That's why community is so important. Each of us can play a part. What can we do? Here are five insights provided by JWRC.

Make a Difference and Lead

When dance teachers intentionally create a positive space where people can grow in community and celebrate what they can do with their body, they do much more than teach dance. They demonstrate safe ways for youth to be in relationships with others. They actively challenge the negative messages abuse survivors have received about their bodies and self-worth. And they actively challenge the messages youth have received either in family or in the media about power and control, especially as the youth watches the teacher use power and authority to lead and help, rather than harm.

Abuse-prevention discussions must become the norm in the dance community. For instance, dance professionals can host occasional seminars for parents, teachers, and community. Ideally, they can join with other studios to host these events. That way, no one risks feeling guilty about "speaking up," and no one fears negative repercussions for their studio. It's expected. It's the norm. Sometimes having a new person on the scene—such as a college intern or a specialist coach—can help the whole studio see things differently.

Parents can lead as well. First, it's important to say something if you have concerns about your child's or any child's safety. Stand up and speak up. Don't assume someone else will.

Parents must also learn to recognize warning signs. Sometimes they're in plain view. Again, offenders take advantage of situations where inappropriate behavior has become normalized.

Is an instructor hugging children too closely and too enthusiastically? Are they touching a child on the upper thigh or carrying the child from one place to another when the child can move on their own? Does the child who loves dance tell their parent, "I don't want to go back there again"? Does the child mention that they're "so good" at dance that they get "special" training with the teacher that no other child receives? Does a studio always follow the "rule of three"—where two adults are present with any interaction with a child?

Finally, parents can help children open up. They shouldn't encourage "secrets" with a child but encourage "surprises." Secrets are when someone doesn't want anyone to find out. That can be confusing to a child, especially when secrets are about safety. But surprises are exciting, and we all know when everyone is going to find out, such as at a surprise birthday party. Then we all can't wait to share.

Model Consent

Dance teachers and parents can set good boundaries by normalizing "asking" before correcting a behavior. For example, a teacher might ask "Can I lift your leg here?" or "Can I show you what I mean by flat back?" rather than just manipulating the child's body without consent. Taking an extra moment to ask and check in with a child or teen helps create a standard where young people know they own their body, whether in or out of class.

For that matter, many adult ballroom dance students can also appreciate and benefit from such courtesies of consent.

Write Policies and Make Them Accessible to Families

Most dance studios have written policies on a wide range of topics, such as clothing, hairstyles, and attendance. But few studios have policies that require training for prevention of abuse and protocols on how to address it. People who cause harm specifically take advantage of this fact. They look for places that don't have policies.

All parents should request to see the child abuse prevention policies. In one case, a mother requested to see the policy and was told, "We don't have policies because we don't hire sex offenders." That's horrifying to hear. We have no way of knowing who sex offenders are. Even background checks hardly help because most abusers are never arrested or convicted.

A written policy makes it easier for parents to speak out if they see something that doesn't seem right. What should policies say? They should document how the studio team invests in safety of students and teachers. The policy should also include best practices, such as requiring two nonrelated adults in the building when open.

In addition, the policy should clarify limitations around texting and social media, usually prohibiting direct text communications between teacher and student without including a parent. Texting and online communications are prime strategies for offenders to groom their targets, with fifteen years old being the average age for online exploitation. Finally, parents and students should know who to contact if they have a safety concern, including an alternate contact if the lead contact is also the person of concern.

When a studio lacks a child abuse prevention policy, parents should at least ask for three dance families to call for references.

Know How to Respond
If You Suspect Abuse

If there's *any* reason to believe that a child is being maltreated, it's important to err on the side of making a report. It's not necessary to interrogate the child. Don't confront the suspected offender because it puts the child at risk. Simply obtain necessary information (names, contacts, and details about suspected behavior), then file a report with police or child protection authorities. It's the adult's responsibility to report, not to investigate.

If a child or teen reveals they're being abused, assure them this is not their fault. Tell them they did the right thing and thank them for telling you. Respect them. Don't have a big reaction, don't be angry with them, and don't pull away from them. Don't make promises except to say, "We'll get more adults involved." Keep the abuse private, not "secret." Then write down the details and call in the report directly.

But again, most children don't disclose abuse. They don't have someone to tell. They don't have the words to explain it. They feel guilty that they may have caused it. They fear being rejected or not believed. Regrettably, 90 percent of children who tell someone have a negative experience telling them.

Parents can help prepare children by having a conversation with them about "what ifs." For example, ask them, "What if your friend was abused? Wouldn't you want someone to know?" Assure your child you just want to make sure they know what to do if something happens, like preparing for a tornado.

Also make sure your child has five adult people they can tell if someone is breaking their own body rules. That raises the chance that at least one of these adults will hear it and take action.

Know Your Resources

In every community, there are people actively involved in addressing child abuse. Get to know your local child advocacy center or other agencies working with families in your community. It's important to have relationships with people doing this important work *before* you need to ask a question or find a resource. Kids are better served when everyone works together to support them.

The Jacob Wetterling Resource Center is one such resource. You can learn more at www.jwrc.org. They also offer a school curriculum called Empower Me, which teaches kids the skills they need to identify and disclose abuse.

The dance community can lead the way in assuring that children have a safe place to express themselves verbally and physically. The skills and experiences children learn through their dance education can protect them for a lifetime.

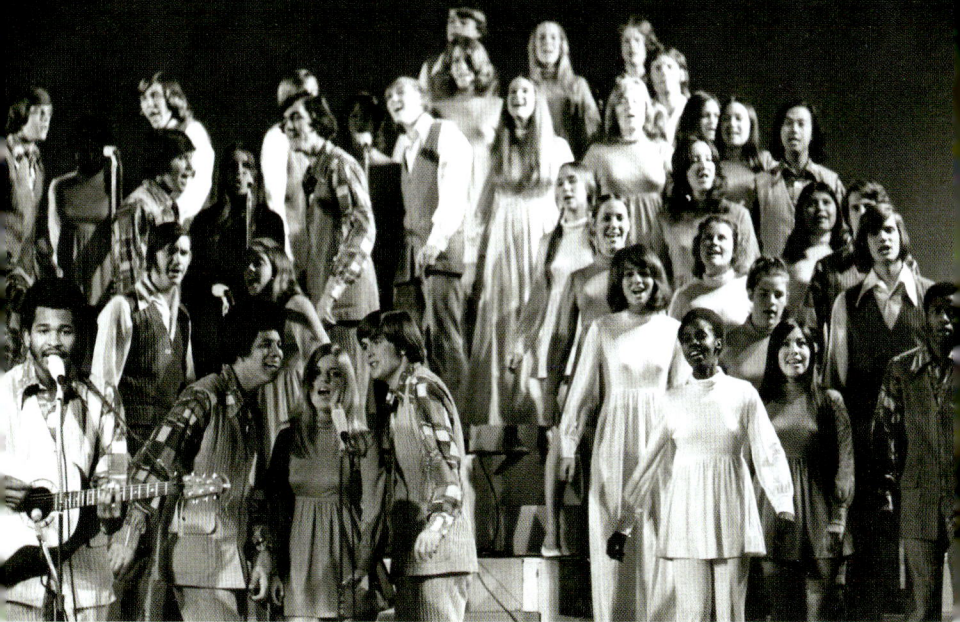
Up with People cast, 1971, Brussels. Ember on microphone facing left, never a dancer. (Chapter 2)

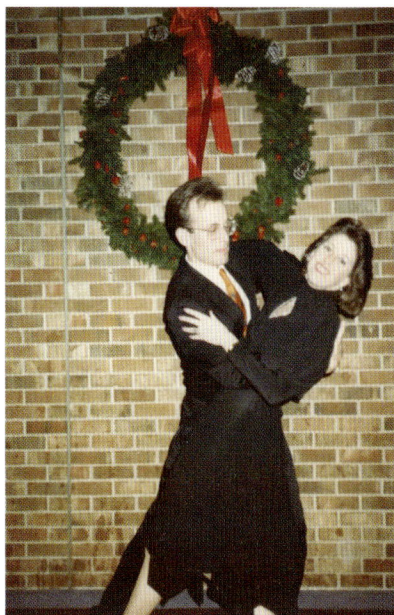
Ember's breakthrough showcase with first instructor John Abrams of Arthur Murray Dance Studios, 1989 (Chapter 2)

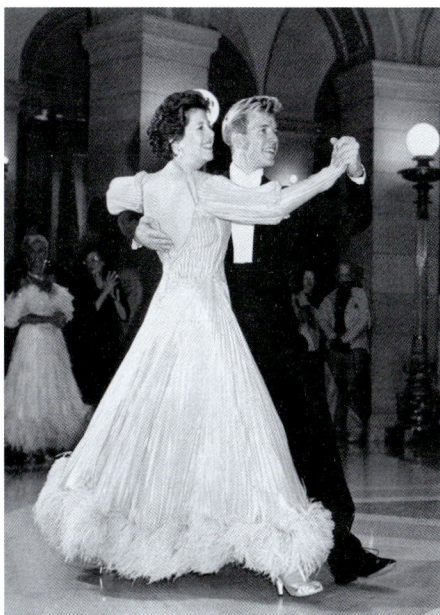
Ember with early Arthur Murray instructor Jesse Smith in Minnesota Capitol rotunda celebrating National Ballroom Dance Week, early 1990s (Chapter 2)

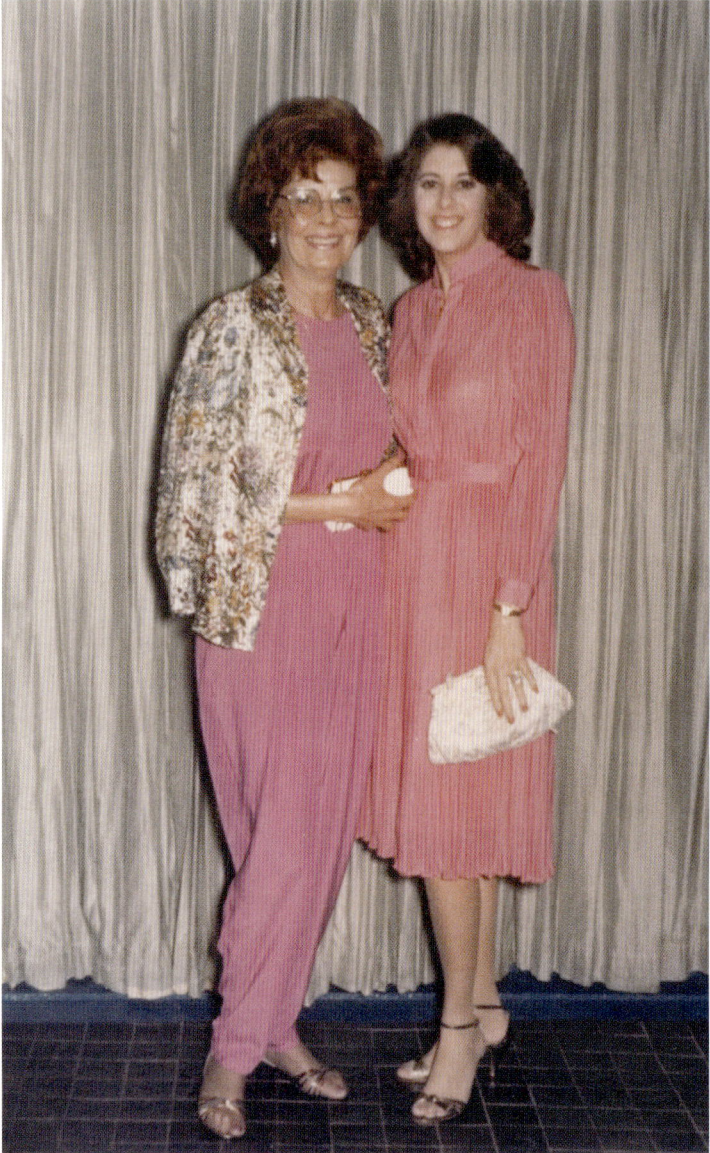

Ember's mom and inspiration, former jitterbug queen Diane Reichgott (Chapter 2)

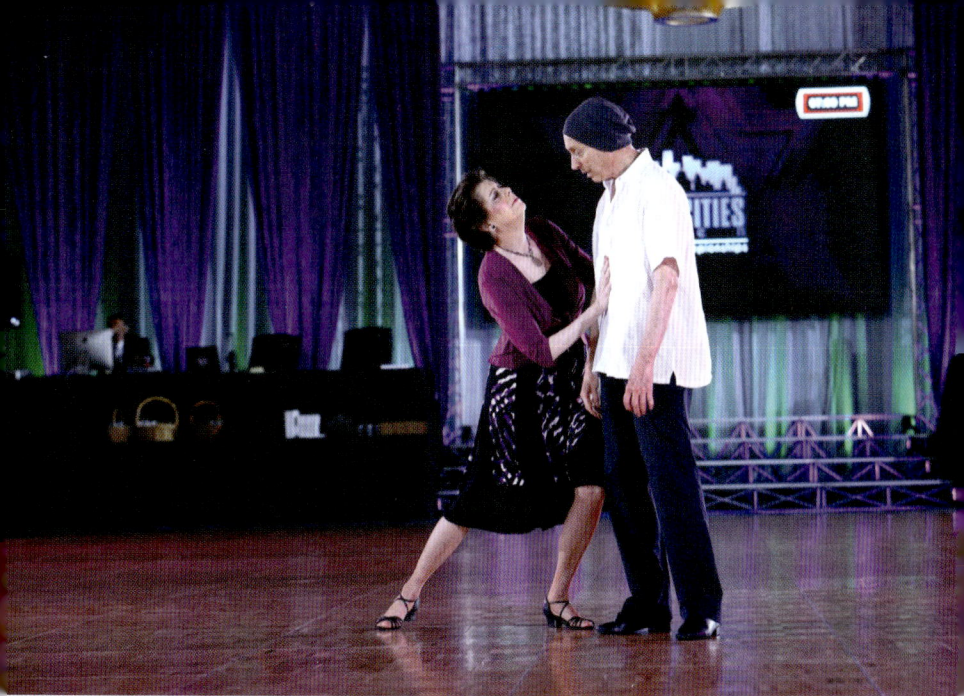

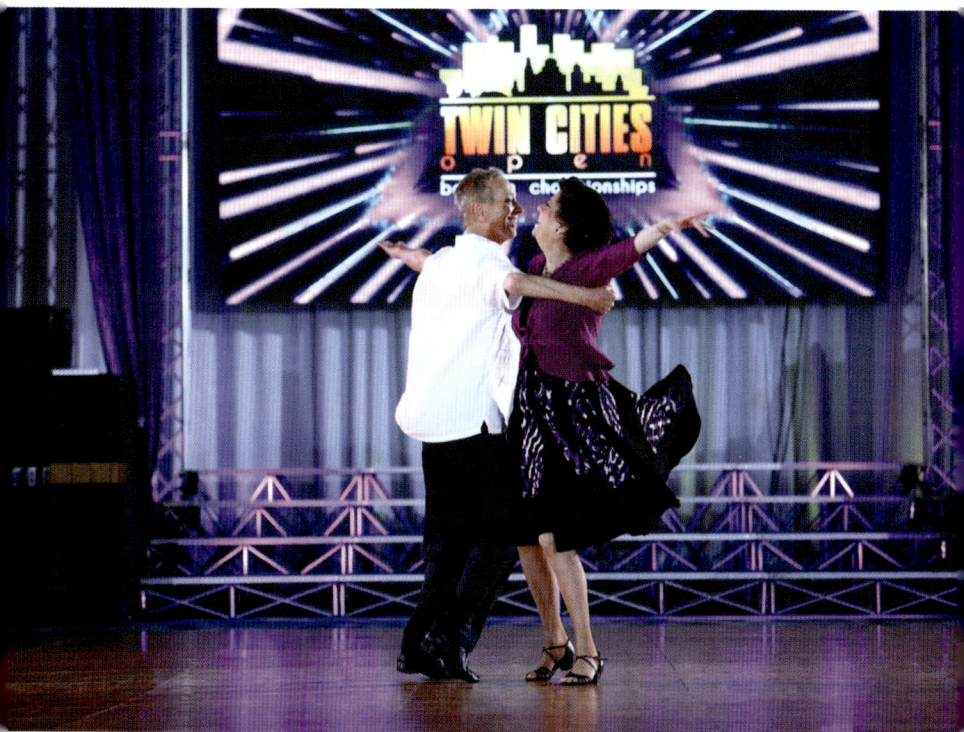

The healing power of dance in Dennis Yelkin's cancer recovery (Chapter 3)

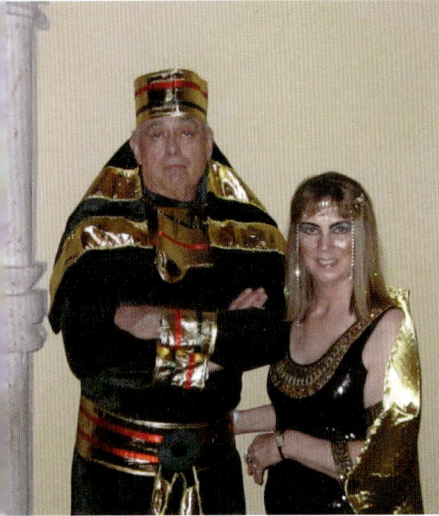

Roger and Melinda Martin
danced till the end. (Chapter 4)

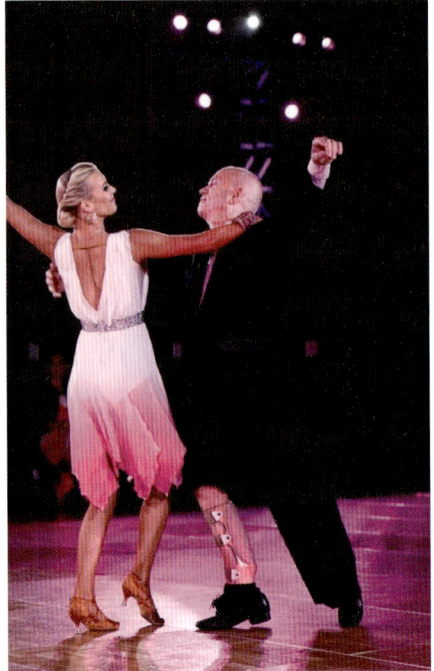

Dr. Paul Cederberg and instructor Meghan Afonkin
(Chapter 6)

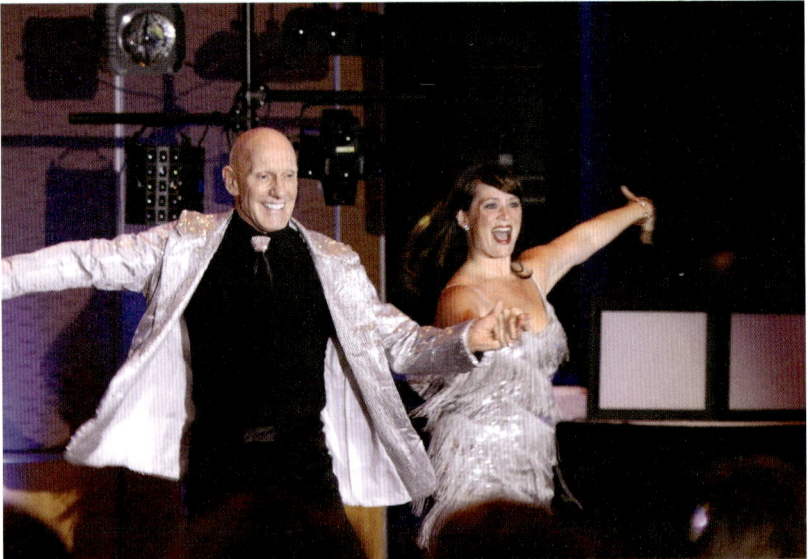

Jim Carter and instructor Andrea Kuzel: "You'll never walk again." (Chapter 5)

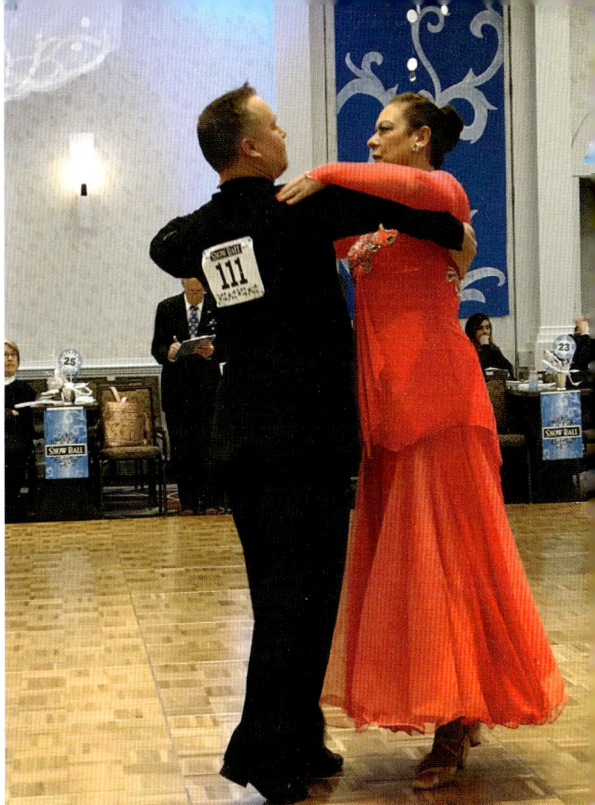

Lisa Davis, who is blind, dancing with instructor Markus Cannon (Chapter 7)

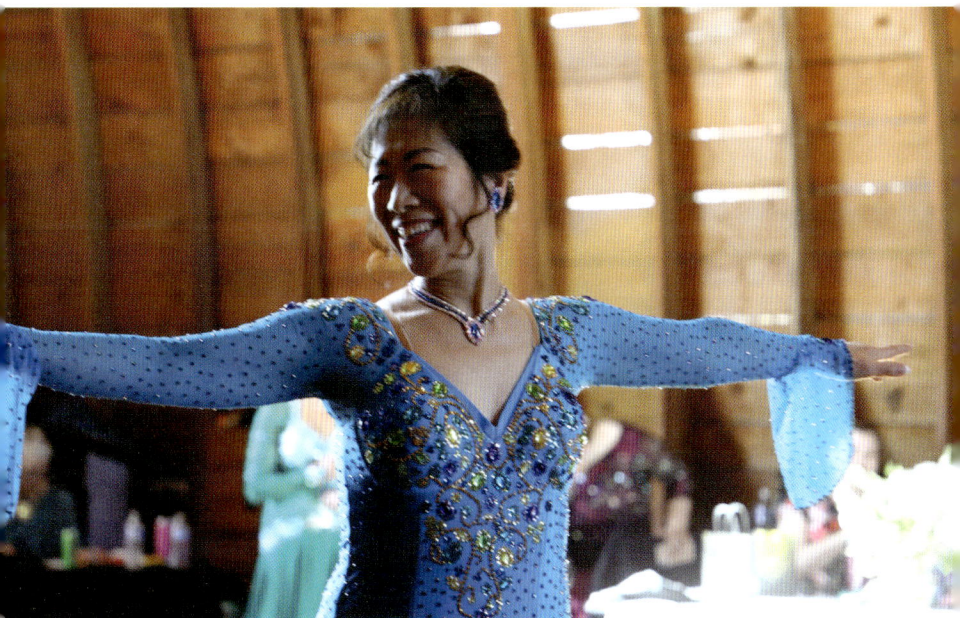

Regina Kim, finding new confidence after emerging from an abusive marriage (Chapter 8)

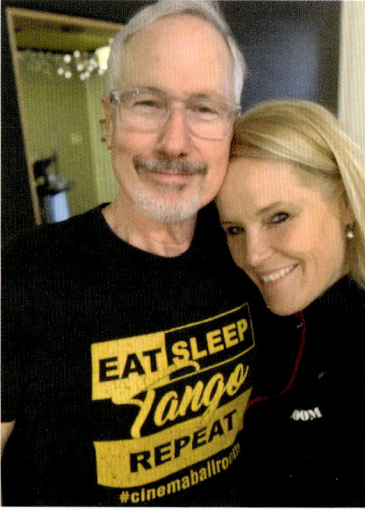

Dan Browning and instructor Michelle Hudson (Chapter 13)

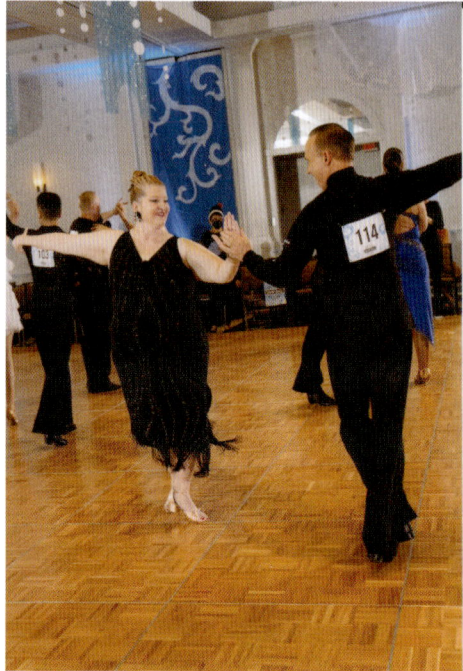

Mike Berman, dancer and political mentor (Chapter 13)

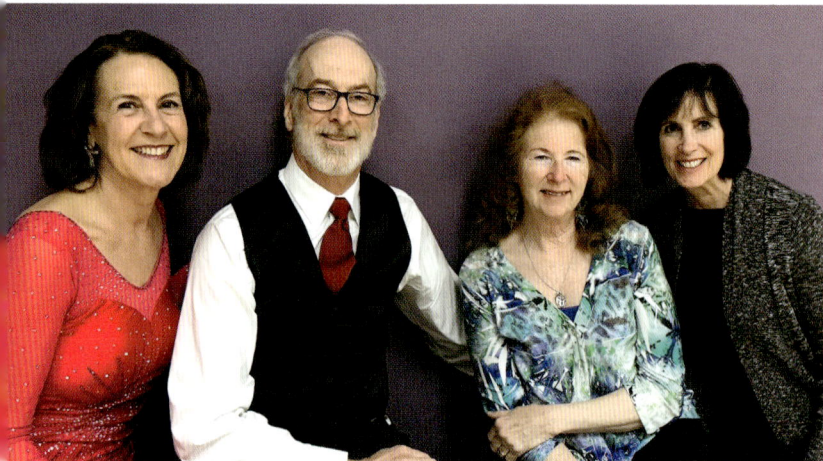

Cindy Snyder rediscovers dance years later with teacher Scott Anderson. (Chapter 11)

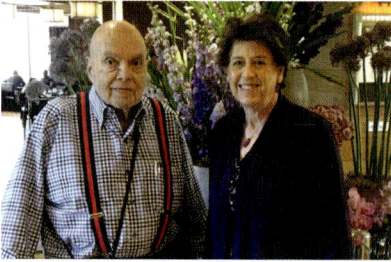

Dr. John Carlson with dance partners Maryann, wife Mary Jo, and Linda (Chapter 12)

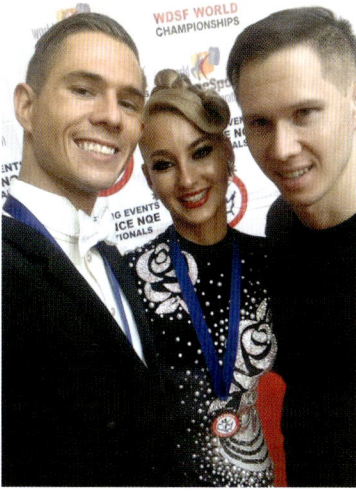

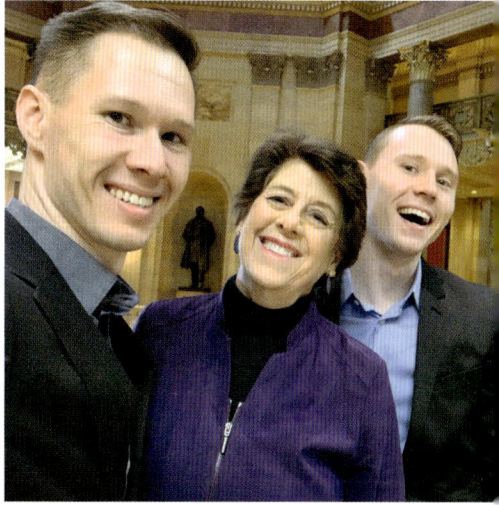

When a light rail crash took Nic Westlake's life and injured fiancée Neli Petkova (left, with medals), brothers Pete and Seth Westlake took action to change a law to prevent future tragedies. (Chapter 14)

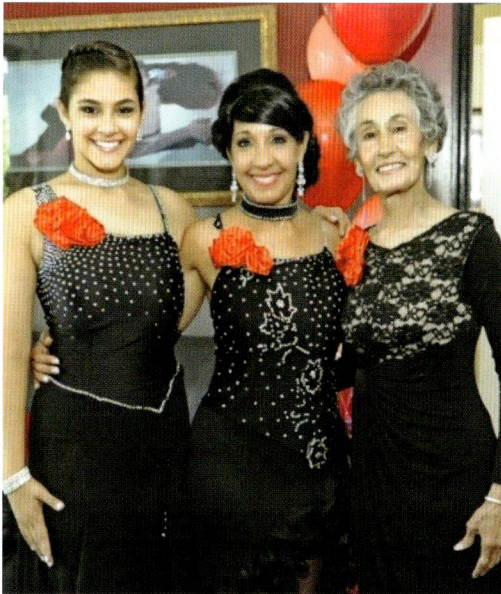

Angela Calabria (right): Never too old to dance; with daughter Alissa Quinn and granddaughter Rachel Quinn (Chapter 15)

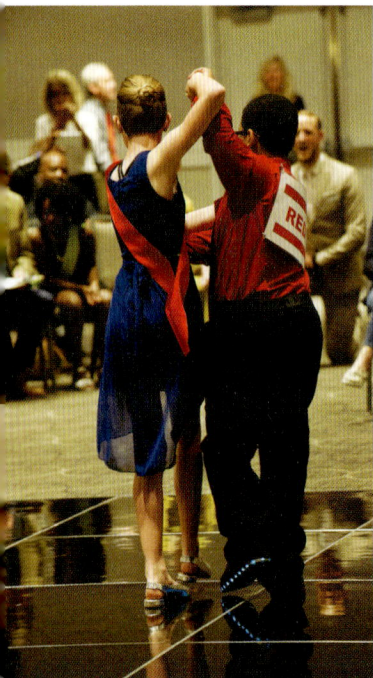

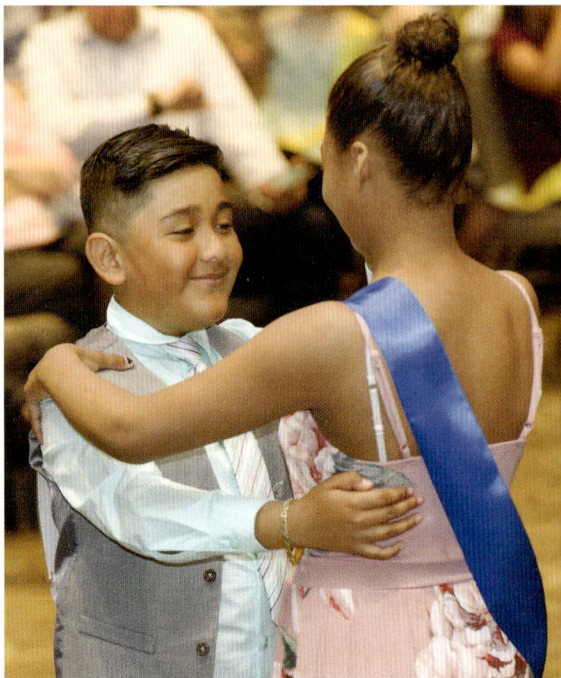

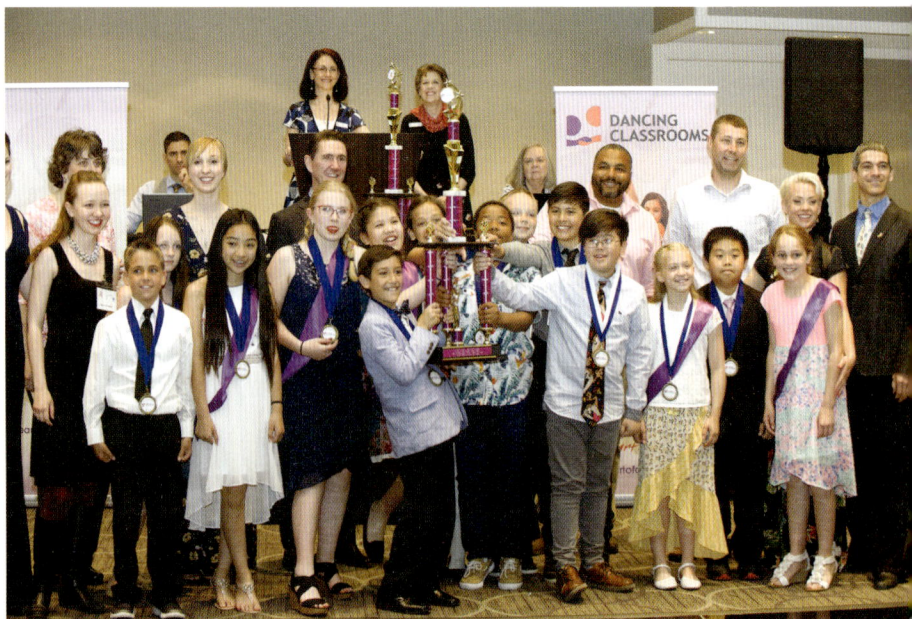

Respect, Teamwork, Elegance: Heart of Dance fifth graders rule! (Chapter 16)

PART III

Relationships: Breaking Down and Breaking Through—Together

Ballroom dance is all about relationships, the key to building resilience in dance and life.

- The relationship between dance teacher and student is intimate in trust, touch, and communication.
- Marriages are created, enriched, and broken through dance. Life partners and dance partners are not always synonymous.
- Some families are built on dance through the generations.

Chapter 18

ﾟ

Dance Coach . . .
or Life Coach?

When people ask ballroom dance professional Nathan Daniels Hawes, "What do you do?" he answers, "I teach life. That's what I do. Dancing is just the vehicle."

The relationship between a ballroom dance teacher and student is like no other. It can be life changing. I know that firsthand.

Think about it. Your teacher is often not your gender. You usually spend at least an hour a week with this person, who is not your romantic partner. You constantly touch—dance is all about touch. It's two bodies moving in sync, sometimes to romantic music. Some dance styles take that to the max, where full body contact is essential throughout.

There has to be trust. That can take years to develop. And it can be emotional. All students learn differently. All teachers teach differently.

There is frustration when you struggle to perform well. There is anxiety as you prepare for a competition or showcase. There is joy when you finally do master something or perform well.

A student may invest time and money for a decade or more with a teacher. A dancer, whether professional or amateur, is never 100 percent accomplished. There are always more techniques to learn and more ways to improve.

And like a bartender or hairstylist, the dance teacher is always there. You've reserved their time, and it's just for you. You have their attention for nearly an hour.

I have poured my heart out to my dance teacher on days when life was hard. His job was to listen and then, somehow, very gently, get me moving. That always helped. I always felt better when I was dancing. Sometimes I have danced out anger. Or it might have been that time of month when the hormones were raging.

Sometimes you share confidences with your teacher and no one else because it's a safe place. The dance teacher deals with all of it. Some are better at this than others. And somehow teachers must control their own issues, desires, and stressors so they can yield to the needs of the students.

It's not always easy. But it's life.

Teachers are valued for their ability to work with students, redirect student frustration, and adjust to unique student needs. This means that the best dance teachers aren't necessarily the best dancers.

Nathan is both.

In one case, Nathan was coaching a couple where the male student was a martial arts expert. His woman partner could not make any sudden move toward him because it would trigger his martial arts training. So Nathan choreographed differently, slowly drawing out her movements to prevent any triggers.

There was also the time when Nathan instructed a woman student to put her arm behind her back. To his surprise, she pulled away sharply and said, "No! That is never going to happen!" Her reaction surprised even her. As it turned out, her past had become her present. She was a survivor of abuse from years before, when she'd been tied up with her arms behind her back.

In another case, Nathan had to adjust to an older student's growing dementia over six years. That was perhaps the most challenging.

"You have to meet them where they are," he said. "You have to pivot all the time."

When working with this student, Nathan created "a whole different skill set" in teaching. He developed a different compassion level, a different way to talk, and a different vocabulary, with certain words he could use or not use. (Find out more in Chapter 28.)

That is life. Dancing is just the vehicle. Again, I know firsthand. Nathan transformed *my* life.

You already know my obsession with perfection when I became a lawyer in my early twenties. I had to be professional at all times. I had to perform exceptionally well so I could become partner in my law firm. God knows, I couldn't make a mistake.

A few years later, I was elected to the Minnesota state senate at age twenty-nine. I was the youngest woman ever elected to that body. The pressure to be professional became more intense, in part because I looked so young. I had to prove that a young woman deserved to be at the statehouse. I was all about "looking good."

I remember attending an early reception near the capitol for an interest group. I took off my coat and boots in the coat room, then turned around to leave. A man proceeded to hand me his coat and boots. When I looked confused, he put two dollars on top. That sure didn't help my confidence.

No wonder I felt I had to be all business. I overprepared everything. Nothing was spontaneous. I didn't know what it felt like to be authentic, to be myself. I was too busy working long hours to achieve my goals, with little time for fun or friends.

Fast-forward a few more years. I was lonely. I was pretty desperate when I walked into that first ballroom dance studio to find a husband. No, I didn't find him right away. But I soon found Nathan, who became my dance teacher.

Coincidently, both Nathan and I had graduated from Duke University in North Carolina. I got my law degree there; he got his undergraduate degree. I found Nathan to be intelligent, well-read, and fascinating. I found his teaching to be direct and no-nonsense. He demanded excellence. When I got frustrated, he would pivot and say something I found hilarious. I liked his sarcasm. Sometimes I doubled over in laughter. Few teachers have that social-emotional skill set.

I developed a deep affection for him and looked forward to my lesson every week. He made me think about things in new ways, well beyond dance.

When I interviewed Nathan for this story, I was prepared to hear how difficult I was as a student, how I always wanted to be in charge. His response surprised me.

"There are certain key things that happen as a teacher when you know you're doing the right thing or you know you've succeeded," Nathan began. "And yours was, 'Nathan, I don't act like this with anyone else but you.' I said, 'What do you mean?' You replied, 'Well, I can just let go and not have to *be* anything. I can be whatever I feel at the moment, whatever I want or need. I can do that because I feel comfortable with you, and you allow me to do that.' So then I was like, 'Well, thank you.' I was just validated."

Validated?

"That's because you were a senator at the time," he said. "You were very in control. You had to be. There was a certain persona and there was a certain attitude and there was a certain command of respect. And when you came to me, it switched because I had to have that role. And it's very hard for a lot of power women to relinquish that control. But I found that when they do, they're much happier people because they can release and they don't have to put on a front. Sometimes you do that just because it's required of your job status."

Nathan paused and turned to me.

"So that's when I knew I was doing the right thing for you. Here was your outlet, where you could just be yourself and not anything else."

Nathan did more than that. He also challenged me to move beyond my comfort zone. I remember how he brought back a fancy Rhythm dress from New York and asked me to wear it for a competition. To me, the tight-fitting dress was downright gaudy, with its shiny silver bodice and bulky black feathers around the thighs. It was way out of my comfort zone—which was probably why I won a top-student award at that competition.

Yes, you nailed it, Nathan. In those weekly dance lessons, I started to discover my playful, authentic self. I was allowing myself to be vulnerable, to learn something new, to make mistakes without the world falling apart, to laugh and have fun. All of that.

Dancing changed me, yes, but in no small part because I had a teacher who understood that challenge and whom I could trust without question. Did it make a difference that he was an African American gay man, someone who was different and nonthreatening in my world? I don't really know. But my life changed forever. And I became the person who met my husband-to-be, Mike, three years later, during summer 1992.

Mike and I married on October 23, 1993. At our wedding reception, Nathan and his professional dance partner, Deanne Michael, generously performed a beautiful showcase dance to our theme song, "Someone Like You." As Nathan lifted Deanne into the air, I thought about how he'd helped lift me from a lonely place to be myself, to love myself, and to love my husband.

Mike and I now celebrate over thirty-two happy years of marriage. And Nathan is a highly respected and admired national dance coach, one of only four male African American ballroom dance judges in the United States.

And yes, I do love Nathan too.

Chapter 19

⌄

Testing Resilience:
Dance Competitions

Participating in a dance competition can bring the highest highs, the lowest lows, the deepest anxieties, or the greatest joys. The small group of ballroom dancers who choose to compete must find their own ways to cope with these emotions. The sport requires intensive preparation and performance.

In the end, it comes down to these things: building resilience, creating unwavering self-confidence, and having a true understanding of yourself. These things are great for dance.

They are even more helpful for life.

The Competition Experience

For me and for many students, the biggest source of emotion—and often frustration—is usually around pro-am ballroom dance competitions, where we as amateur students dance with our professional teachers. That may be the most difficult frustration for teachers to manage.

These competitions are a world of their own. Imagine a huge, brightly lit hotel ballroom filled with dance teachers and their elegantly dressed students twirling around a crowded dance floor, their faces sometimes locked in plastic smiles as a panel of judges observe from the edges of the floor. The gentlemen dancers, wearing numbers safety-pinned to the backs of their formal jackets or glitzy shirts, dance full-out as they work to avoid bumping other dancers traveling at high speed just feet away.

Nearly every week, there is a ballroom dance competition happening somewhere in the United States and beyond. The competitions include every style imaginable, from traditional ballroom styles to nightclub, country, and Argentine tango.

Competition is not for everyone, though. Of all the ballroom dancers in the world, only a small percentage compete. And an even smaller cohort compete at the more advanced levels.

Why do we do it?

For many dancers, occasional competitions are a fun way to improve their dancing. Remember Cindy Snyder, the former dance teacher you met in Chapter 11, who returned to dance years later as an amateur student? I loved how she described competitions as pageants.

"It's a fun outlet, where everybody gets to be all dolled up and dressed up," she said. "They get to be ladies and gentlemen. They get to treat each other nicely. It's such a departure from society right now."

Amen.

For Cindy, competitions aren't about "competing" at all. They're about improving.

"I think you have to compare yourself to yourself," she said. "You look at your scores and compare to how you did the last time or the last dance, and you try to improve from there. I don't think it's me against somebody else. It's more about myself against myself. That's where the benefit of competition lies."

I've said before that the community aspect of ballroom dance is important to me. That's become even more true in competitions as I've grown older. I love dancing in Minnesota competitions because dancers from studios all over the state are there. They cheer me on, and I cheer them on. We all try to do our best. We're among friends. More and more, I've been engaging in deeper conversations to know and respect them as whole persons, not just dancers. It opens a whole new world of connecting. I love it.

Yes, community draws me into more competitions, perhaps because when you are with good friends, you also discover more about yourself. Self-discovery now occurs every time I compete. That potential breakthrough somehow outweighs my other emotions that inevitably arise from competition.

Of course, that's just me. Every dancer is different. For some, there's the fun and excitement of traveling around the country to practice your chosen passion in various competitions.

Patrick Moriarity loves this aspect. A stocky and rounded amateur dancer now in his seventies, Pat has danced with several women ballroom dance instructors in numerous competitions over thirteen years.

Pat is not the first person you'd expect to be a dancer. Pat took his first dance lesson only because he lost a bet with a coworker. As Eric Hudson, owner of Cinema Ballroom, once said, "If you were to select for a high school yearbook the person 'Least likely to become a ballroom dancer,' that would be Pat Moriarity."

Here's the proof: One time, Pat and Nadine Messenger, his professional instructor from Cinema Ballroom, mistakenly arrived at the Minneapolis–Saint Paul airport five hours late for their flight to a dance competition. They begged the ticket agent to book them as quickly as possible on the next flight to Las Vegas, explaining that they needed to get to a ballroom dance competition.

The ticket agent looked over the portly, gray-haired sixty-five-year-old gentleman with the sexy twenty-year-old lady at his side. Nadine was dressed to the hilt. The agent wasn't buying the story and wanted nothing to do with them. She sent them off to customer service.

"I think she thought Nadine was a Vegas working girl," Pat said. "And the way Nadine was dressed, I could understand that."

So Pat and Nadine went to the customer service area and begged to get on the next flight. But the reservationist had a similar reaction to the couple. She didn't buy their story about needing to get to a dance competition.

Finally, the reservationist asked, "Can you dance here?"

Pat and Nadine set their belongings down and moved to the center of the floor. Pat raised his arm to invite Nadine to dance. With elegant frame, they danced their choreographed waltz routine in the middle of the Delta customer service area. About thirty people waiting in the area were entertained with delight, showing their appreciation with whistling and applause.

The reservationist watched from behind the counter. When they finished, she said, "You just earned yourself a ticket on the flight you wanted."

It's one of Pat's most memorable dance experiences.

Battling Competition Demons

The competitive aspect of dance competitions can be difficult, of course. The right attitude is important.

But for most, emotions rule.

You remember Greta Anderson from Chapter 10, the young woman who froze and nearly walked away from her first ballroom dance lesson with teacher Gordon Bratt. Greta's confidence grew as she experienced success in her dance career. In 2018, she started traveling to out-of-state competitions, winning first in her division at the prestigious Emerald Ball national competition.

"I went up to my room and cried, I was so happy," Greta recalled.

But then she didn't do so well at another competition, and that was another crucible for her.

"I remember going home and thinking, 'You can either be done, let this take you out, sulk about your placements, or you can say *You wrote off the wrong girl!* and go back and fight.' That's part of the challenge. You can't blame the judges or others for your defeat. You have to look inward for what more you can do. What do you need to change? When you pour your heart and soul into something, and you're met with defeat, that's not an easy pill to swallow. But it's a competition—it has to happen to someone."

This is the battle of resilience that I've personally fought throughout my dance career. I'm an achiever. Always have been. In fact, Achiever is one of my top five Strengths according to the popular CliftonStrengths assessment. That means I like to set goals and achieve them.

It explains my drive. Every day, I need to achieve something tangible or complete an important task to feel satisfied. If I accomplish my goal, it feels good for a short time, but then my need to achieve rekindles itself, pushing me toward my next accomplishment.

The Achiever strength pushes me forward in dance. I'll work like crazy to learn a new technique that I believe will help me be better. I get energy from that. As Clifton describes, "It is the jolt you can always count on to get you started on new tasks, new challenges."

But the Achiever strength is a double-edged sword. If I set a goal in a competition (to place in the finals, for example) but I don't achieve that goal, the emotions flow. Especially if I danced well and performed the new techniques that I learned.

Over the years, I've placed first in multi-dance fields, and I've placed last—sometimes in the same competition! Placing last is, of course, the most difficult for me to reconcile. I didn't achieve anything, did I? That "Unreasonable Fear of Making a Mistake" (and being ashamed or embarrassed) comes back in full force. *How could I have danced that way in front of all those people? I'm sure I embarrassed my instructor and our studio. I've been dancing a long time. People expect me to do better.*

Or maybe no one actually cared. And maybe I did achieve something—maybe I danced better than ever but against a more experienced field. These are reasonable perspectives, but my head doesn't necessarily go there.

So when I first embarked on my dance competition journey, my initial struggle was to develop the resilience to overcome these emotions. I had to learn how to recognize my improvements and achievements regardless of where I placed in a competition, like my friend Cindy described. I had to learn how to move on to the next improvement, the next achievement, whether it showed up in the next competition.

I danced some enjoyable Bronze- and early-Silver-level years with Nathan Daniels, including in competitions. I attended my first out-of-state competition with him in Las Vegas. It felt like the "big leagues" to me!

In the mid-1990s, I moved on to instructor Scott Anderson and had a good experience overall. I was doing well in placements.

But as you learned in Chapter 13, I then stopped dancing entirely around 1997. For a long time.

Like about fourteen years.

As I shared earlier, I told myself that I'd stopped dancing because my responsibilities in the senate were increasing and because I was seeking a higher statewide office. When my 1998 campaign for attorney general was unsuccessful, I chose to retire from the Minnesota Senate in 2001, completing eighteen years of service. And as I also shared, I was grieving the loss of both my parents, two other close family members, and my best friend—all of which happened in less than five years.

Through all this, it didn't occur to me to return to dance to help manage my emotions. That seems strange, given how much I loved dance and the impact it made on my life. Dance could have served me well.

Writing a book like this is about self-discovery. As I look back all these years later, I think I better understand why I *really* left dance and didn't return for so many years.

I recall dancing in a competition in St. Louis with teacher Scott Anderson; it was my last competition before I stopped dancing. I also recall—with a fresh twinge—the heartbreak I felt when I didn't make the finals in either of my dance categories.

I was far from achieving my goals. It was painful.

I suspect now that stopping dance was my way to end the pain. With all that was going on in my life, I just didn't have the strength, resilience, or emotional wherewithal to understand my pain or overcome it.

So I stopped. For fourteen years.

What ultimately brought me back, in 2011? Another passion, perhaps even stronger than dance.

As a legislator, I led efforts in the senate to prevent family violence and child sexual abuse. One day, I received a call from the executive director of CornerHouse, a nonprofit organization I'd worked with that supports survivors of child sexual abuse and trains law enforcement and others how to identify and prosecute perpetrators of sexual abuse. The director asked if I would be a "celebrity" dancer in their annual Let's Dance fundraiser.

That was all I needed. I dusted off my dance shoes, began lessons again, and performed a foxtrot to "New York, New York" with dance instructor Chris Kempainen, who generously volunteered his time. It got my Achiever instincts going because it was not only a chance to dance again but also a chance to fundraise for a great cause. At the time, I was the chief advancement officer for Lutheran Social Service of Minnesota, so I definitely knew how to raise money. I was named champion with Chris and was invited to return two more years, once again with Chris and later with Scott Anderson.

The CornerHouse fundraisers brought back the joy of dance to my life. They also brought a different joy—the joy of performing before an audience of people who were *not* ballroom dancers. Part of my enjoyment was the chance to inspire others to enjoy ballroom dance, which had been so important in my life. Several friends I met through that experience took up dancing for themselves. *Yes!*

I think that experience planted the seeds for the purpose of this book.

Competition Demons:
What the Dance Pros Say

With time, I've come to realize that many factors come into play for competitive dancing—factors dancers often do not control. Professional instructors can best describe those factors.

My former instructor Nathan Daniels recalls when he and his professional partner Deanne Michael were frustrated because they were "working their asses off" yet their competition placements were not going up.

Their coach, Eddie Simon, responded, "Nathan, do you think those other people aren't working hard too? They may be working even harder than you are, believe it or not. You have time restraints and parameters, and maybe they don't. Deanne has a baby, maybe they don't. Get over yourself. Just do what you do, and it will happen."

That put things in perspective for Nathan—a perspective he has gone on to share with his students. When they ask, "Why didn't I win?" Nathan tells them, "You have no control over your winning. All you have control over is how you dance and what you put out there. You could dance the same exact way five different times and get five different results because the judging panel is different or because they're looking at you at different times. You looked unsure here, and you were great over there, but they didn't see that great thing, only the insecure part."

Nathan is now a dance judge himself, which means he sees the other side of this perspective. He turns this experience into advice for his students as well.

"You can't go out to 'beat' someone," he said. "That's never going to happen. If you do place ahead, that's great. But the odds are, if someone gets coaching two hours a week, and someone else gets it five hours a week, the person getting five hours will probably do better just because they put more time and energy into it. Also, the more you compete, the better your results will probably be because coaching can't replicate competition floor time. There's a certain comfort level with people who compete all the time, compared to people who may be more talented but only compete two or three times a year. There's a different look on the floor. They just feel comfortable. They look more natural. It just happens."

One thing Nathan understands as a dancer, teacher, and judge is that hard work is a given.

"There are people who say, 'I want to be a champion.' Well, everyone wants to be a champion. But few people are really willing to do what it takes to be a champion. You have to have time, energy, money, and desire. You also have to have some talent. But the most talented people are not the ones who usually win. It's the ones who have the most drive and ambition. Talent is a very small part of it. Some very talented people don't work hard enough because they know they're talented and it comes easy to them. But they're never going to be a champion because they don't have the same drive."

I hear this from other professional dance teachers. Gene Bersten is one—you'll meet him and his family later in this Part III. Gene and his younger brother, Alan, were both national Latin champions in the junior and youth divisions, and Alan is currently a celebrity professional on *Dancing with the Stars*. Gene is currently competing and winning national competitions with his wife, Elena.

"Some may say we're talented," Gene said. "But I say talent means nothing in this industry. It's all about hard work. The harder worker will always pass the more talented dancer. Talent, of course, helps. It gives you a head start. But the hard work— the technique, the foundation—will always shine through."

But even hard work sometimes isn't enough. To Gene, it's also about having confidence in yourself. When Gene coached Alan during their younger years, Gene talked with him before every competition to motivate him in the right way.

"My brother and I are very competitive," Gene said. "It's a mind-set. We're competitors. If we want to win, we first have to win in our heads. If you have any self-doubt, it always comes out when you're dancing. I always do this with my students too. I want them to feel nervous in the lesson, not at the competition."

Remember those CliftonStrengths I mentioned? I suspect Gene has Competition as one of his Strengths. According to the original *Now, Discover Your Strengths* book by Marcus Buckingham and Donald Clifton, Competition is rooted in comparison. Other people's performance is the ultimate yardstick. "You like contests because they must produce a winner," Buckingham and Clifton write. "Although you are gracious to your fellow competitors and even stoic in defeat, you don't compete for the fun of competing. You compete to win."

Growing Resilience in Competitions

No matter one's strengths, most dancers at any level will find competitions to be a bit of a roller coaster. Resilience allows you to find ways to not get down on yourself—and not quit for fourteen years, like I did.

Now older and perhaps wiser, I keep coming back to dance. That may be the most important demonstration of my resilience. Today I marvel at the benefits dance has brought to me and my dance colleagues.

I especially recognized these benefits during the COVID pandemic, when all I could do was sit home and write stories about dancing. During that time, I missed all that dancing had brought to my life.

I've also come to realize that competitions are benchmarks, not goals. That has become clear as I've danced through my late sixties and into my seventies.

I continue to build acceptance and gratitude for how far I've come and for how much joy I've gained from this experience. But acceptance doesn't necessarily mean approval. I don't have to "approve" everything I've danced, and the judges don't have to either. But I do need to accept what I've done. It is what it is.

Acceptance frees me up to set my next goal and continue my drive to improve. I want—and *need*—to improve. That's the Achiever strength in me. I don't necessarily need to win; that's more like the Competition strength. But I need to know and recognize my improvement. And yes, I also need my teacher and dance colleagues to acknowledge it as well.

I need to know that what I'm doing in my dance practice is *productive*. I work hard. So if I don't do well, I need to understand what's missing, what I'm not doing, and what I must do to improve next time.

Understanding is sometimes elusive. Some teachers are better than others at breaking down your competition videos and then identifying and teaching the techniques or tweaks you need to work on. I like when teachers do that. My current instructor, Martin Pickering of Cinema Ballroom, does that well. It works for me, and it gets me on my way again. But if I don't understand or if the teacher is not adept at explaining the "why," it's pure frustration for me. I don't know how to improve.

We all learn differently. And good teachers adjust to the learning needs of their students. I suggest that both dance teachers and students assess their personal strengths through the Clifton-Strengths assessment and use that guidance to better understand each other. It works. And not just for dance partners.

From the Therapist Who Dances: Finding Calm

This is just my personal experience, for sure. Yours will be different. But can we generalize some lessons for others, both in dance and in life?

I turned to my good friend Angie Star. She has been ballroom dancing for five years with my instructor, Martin Pickering. She and I share a special bond: We each traveled worldwide for a year (though fifteen years apart) with the international musical cast of Up with People.

Angie has been a therapist in social work and psychotherapy since 1990. Today she calls herself a coach. For her, dance is not just a physical journey but a mental and emotional one. She poses the broader question of *Can we make room for that?*

We can get stuck in our dance journey as we try to overcome fears and blocks. Yes, our dance journey will bring things up. Can we have the courage to face these obstacles, to be curious, and to learn something about ourselves? Do we have the courage to face our blocks and understand them, instead of trying to push them out of the way?

I can attest to the effectiveness of Angie's coaching model, rooted in Internal Family Systems (IFS). Maybe you can too. She summarizes it simply as "What part of you is in the driver's seat?" We all have "parts"—patterns, personalities, tendencies. And we all have our authentic "Self." But who's running the show?

First, Angie counsels that we need to appreciate that our body is a better dancer than our brain. Our brain really wants to help, and we can appreciate that. But sometimes our brain works too hard, and it overthinks everything and gets in the way.

Sometimes we need to trust our body over our brain. That is, we need to trust our body memory. In order for this to work, we need to give our brain just *one* thing to think about so it can relax and let our body dance.

"If I don't focus on one thing, my brain will grab twenty things," Angie explained. "That focus allows me to be more connected to my body and the music. Ultimately, the dancing is more enjoyable. I'll know when my brain is working too hard. The round of dance will feel off."

So how does Angie get into a good headspace for competition?

"I don't over-practice. I'm in touch with my nervous system. I'm paying attention to my parts. I need to know and feel confident in the choreography—that's one part. But it's just as important to me to be calm. I just dance better when I'm calm. That takes effort. I put as much effort into being calm as I do into practicing. We think a competition is all about practicing and being on top of your game, but for me, it's a bigger picture than that."

Angie tries to maintain self-compassion—compassion for the parts of her that tend to get scared. The reality, however, is that some parts don't *want* to be compassionate.

"I encourage people to find a mind-set of curiosity toward themselves instead of accepting 'I just get so nervous,'" she said. "What is it about competitions that brings up fear? I encourage people to have the courage to be honest with themselves. 'What am I afraid of?'"

Sometimes fear comes from a part of the brain that sees competition as a threat. Angie demonstrates how we can explore and diffuse that.

"Am I unconsciously seeing the judges as a threat? Am I afraid of disappointing my teacher? Am I afraid of disappointing myself? I encourage clients to have the courage to get underneath that fear and not just accept it. What if you don't have to be afraid? If you don't want to be anxious at competitions, you must make room for the possibility that it doesn't have to be this way."

Lastly, Angie encourages dancers to set goals and not give themselves mixed messages.

"If I practice, practice, practice in response to being anxious, what goal am I trying to achieve? My goal is not to be perfect in my dancing. My goal is to be calm. The goal of being perfect, I think, creates anxiety. And if I practice, practice, I will feed it. So the real issue is being clear about your goal and being aware of any unconscious goals you may have."

How lucky I am to have a good friend who is a therapist! Her counsel on a long car ride to a recent competition helped me rediscover my calm. I danced better than ever.

And what awareness did I uncover along the way? That those high expectations my mother instilled in me years ago may well be part of my unconscious goals. I can appreciate that I have those high expectations. But I don't want them to be in my driver's seat. I get to decide. I can decide that I will hold those expectations in check.

Today, I still set competition goals, but they don't rule my dance life. Competitions are more fun now. I love to dance.

I love to perform. You don't have to be a champion dancer to bring joy to yourself and others.

This type of acceptance is even more helpful as you age. Ironically, the senior level pro-am categories can be some of the most populated and competitive in the ballroom world.

I feel so fortunate to have the health, cognitive ability, and resources to dance and to occasionally compete at my stage in life. It brings me such reward and satisfaction. That should be all I need, and I work hard every day to accept and celebrate that.

This book and its mission to inspire others to dance into their mature years help me do that every day.

Chapter 20

✔

Enriching Marriage
Through Dance

A marriage and a dance partnership are two very different relationships. There are similarities, of course. Both relationships are usually long-term, requiring significant time in the other's presence. Communication can be intense, and it's easy to trigger emotions.

So imagine the tensions that can result when the two relationships overlap. Sometimes marriage and dance partnerships work in combination. Other times, they don't. Either way, it can build a new kind of resilience.

The following three couples generously shared their experiences at different stages (and outcomes) of dance and marriage. One commonality binds them all: Spouses who dance learn new skills that enhance both their individual lives as well as their partnership.

Waltzing into Midlife Marriage

You marry early in life, have kids, and start your careers. By the time your kids head to college, you're accomplished in your careers, and you've settled into your marital routine. What now?

Try starting *serious* ballroom dancing with your spouse!

That's what Scott and Bernie Osborn did. For them, it was a real "high."

"Dancing gave us a feeling of belonging to a wonderful new group of people," Bernie said. "It was the beginning of a whole new phase of married life."

Their friends Art and Cheri Rolnick made the same decision. For them, dancing added so much.

"It enriched our lives, our communication, and our marriage," Cheri said.

When the two middle-aged couples started free social dance classes with professional Jeff Nehrbass at their local fitness club, dance wasn't entirely new to any of them. As Le Sueur High School sweethearts, Scott and Bernie had enjoyed swing and slow dances together at prom and elsewhere. (Scott: "I thought she was hot!") Art had taken social dance lessons in Detroit so he could dance at his bar mitzvah. Cheri was a self-described "street dancer," later encouraged by her future mother-in-law to successfully audition as a go-go dancer.

Today, both couples celebrate more than fifty years of marriage and their roles as grandparents, plus they've danced at the highest levels of amateur ballroom dance competition and are still dancing together in their seventies. They recently retired from over twenty-five years on a high-level dance formation team, where my partner and I enjoyed dancing regularly with them as teammates for about five years.

Getting Started

"I had no idea what I was getting into with dancing," Bernie said. "No idea. I just wanted to dance. But it's not that easy. You have to start at the beginning. It's a lot more involved than I thought."

Bernie worked in banking and later in school administration, but her urge to dance stretched back to her childhood.

"I grew up on a farm with ten siblings," she said. "You didn't always get to do what you wanted. Dance was one of those things for me. I always had a deep interest in it."

Dr. Scott Osborn, who owned a dental practice before his retirement, added, "My dental patients would tell me 'That's so romantic!' when they heard I was a ballroom dancer. No! If you're going to do competitive dance, it is anything *but* romantic! It's a lot of work."

The Osborns began by taking private Bronze-level lessons from Jeff and Cindy Nehrbass. Bronze is the first level of competitive dance and is more technical and formulaic than social dance. A dancer usually masters the Bronze level before moving on to the Silver and Gold competition levels. But things don't always go as planned.

At an early showcase, Bernie and Scott were set to perform their Bronze waltz routine. But the stress of performing in front of people caused Scott to unexpectedly lead Silver-level steps, causing a bit of a meltdown.

"Don't ever make me do this again!" he told Bernie as they came off the floor.

"Jeff came over," Bernie recalled. "He said, 'What in hell were you doing out there?' Scott replied, 'What can I say? I panic in Silver.'"

There seems to be an independent streak in middle-aged beginners. When Art and Cheri started taking lessons with Jeff, they insisted on starting at the Gold level. Did Jeff agree with that?

"No!" Cheri said with a laugh. "We didn't listen to him. He also told us not to start by competing at a national competition, but that's where we first competed. We didn't know what we were doing. Art was dancing every which way. In the middle of heats, a judge pulled me off and asked, 'Do you know about line of dance?' 'What does that mean?' I asked. He said, 'See this circle? Try to stay in it.'"

"We were such novices, but we had fun," Art added. "We actually got first place because there were no other competitors with us in the Gold level."

This independent streak may arise in part because both Rolnicks have doctorate degrees. Dr. Cheri Rolnick is an epidemiologist who once worked with Dr. Anthony Fauci on a major AIDS grant and later became associate director of research at the Health Partners Foundation.

"My career as an epidemiologist used my intellect," said Cheri, "but music touches my soul."

And Dr. Art Rolnick was the director of research for the Federal Reserve Bank of Minneapolis. For him, dance wasn't about the soul but the mind.

"When we first started taking coaching lessons," he said, "I kind of pooh-poohed it intellectually. I figured it's no big deal. Then I realized how intellectual it was. The coaches were amazing. You had to understand body movement and coordination and choreography. I like the intellectual aspect of it. I found the coaches to be really bright people, and I enjoyed interacting with them—not just about dancing but the social aspect of it."

Today the Rolnicks still work with professionals Nathan Daniels and Mariusz Olszewski.

Formation Team: The Equalizer

Key to the dance development of both couples was their early participation in a dance formation team initially organized by Nehrbass and later by Scott Anderson and Deanne Michael.

"I'd asked Jeff to do this for some time," Bernie said. "I like dancing with our friends on the floor. I'm a bit anxious, so this makes competitions less nerve-racking and a lot more fun."

Her husband, Scott, added, "The formation helped us with technique that we used in our individual dancing."

Both the Osborns and the Rolnicks loved the social aspects of the formation team.

"It's a great equalizer," Art said. "When you're on the dance floor, they don't care if you're a CEO, a plumber, an educator, or a billionaire. They just care about dancing. We've met wonderful people through dancing that we would never have met socially."

"We made some really close friends," Scott agreed. "There were probably one hundred members of the team on and off, over twenty-five years. The teams brought all kinds of people together from all walks of life."

As an example, the Osborns hired a fellow dance member to improve the landscape of their yard and became dear friends with him.

The formation team was pivotal for the Rolnicks in another way. Since all the other couples were dancing in competitions, the Rolnicks had to take private weekly lessons to keep up. Art didn't want to compete, but Jeff taught them routines anyway.

Then Cheri was invited to compete in a national competition with another professional partner, in part due to her small size because the routine included lifts. Art decided to go to the competition with her. So why not get on the dance floor themselves? Hence, that first national competition at the Gold level.

And the rest is history.

Taking the "Lead" in Marriage and Dance

There's no doubt that bringing dance into marriage (or marriage into dance?) requires a strong foundation and communication. This was the case for the Osborns and the Rolnicks. Each couple was so connected that one spouse could hardly start a thought without the other finishing it. In addition, they weren't shy about their strengths and weaknesses.

"I think ballroom dancing is like life in general," Scott began. "You have good days. Bad days. Days when you're upset with each other. Days when things are going beautifully. And in some ways, ballroom dancing is like golf," he added. "If you're a mediocre golfer, you hit just enough good shots to keep you coming back to the game, right? Well, when you have a dance that feels so effortless, and when you walk off the floor and you know you've just nailed it, it's a high. It's a great feeling. As in life, it doesn't happen all the time."

And when it doesn't happen, what does it feel like?

Bernie said, "I imagine that everyone has some tension in dancing when you're face-to-face with your partner. And if you're married, you tend to be a little more . . ."

"It's easier to express yourself," Scott finished.

"Through the years, I've learned to let go a lot quicker," Bernie said. "Because it's dancing, and we love it, but we've just got to . . ."

"Keep in mind why you're doing it," Scott chimed in again. "A lot of times, the husband and wife have different interests and spend many hours apart. We decided to do something together."

And how did the couple handle frustrations on the dance floor?

"One thing that hit home for me a lot is that if things weren't going well, it was usually the leader that was the problem," Scott said.

"I love hearing that!" Bernie quickly added.

"Being a dentist and a perfectionist, it's hard to admit to being the person at fault," Scott continued. "But when you learn the problem and how to correct it, that makes it that much better. Most dentists are perfectionists. But when that carries over to your personal life, that can be a real problem for the other person."

"I have different needs than him," Bernie said. "He caught on real quick!"

One thing the Osborns found helpful after several decades of male coaches was working with a woman coach, Meghan Anderson Afonkin.

"From my perspective," Scott said, "Meghan has an uncanny ability to diagnose the problem with the lead. She would coach me through it. She would 'back lead' me so I knew how it was supposed to feel. When I went back to dance with Bernie, nine times out of ten she was smiling because she could feel the difference."

"Trying to figure that out as an amateur couple," Bernie said, "you really can't do it . . ."

"Especially if one of us is a perfectionist and we think we know it all!" Scott added.

The lead was also the key issue for Art and Cheri.

"The tension comes because the man has to lead and the woman has to follow," Art said. "Coaches would tell Cheri, 'You live for the lead.' She'd say, 'Fine. Where is the lead?'"

Over the years, the couple has learned to negotiate. When they learn choreography, Art first concentrates on his part and practices a long time. He tells Cheri, "Lead yourself. Don't expect anything from me." Then when he feels more confident, he announces, "I'm ready to lead."

This is tough for Cheri. "I catch on to dance much more quickly than Art. Our learning styles are so very different. I feel the music—the music talks to me."

"She's more natural," Art agreed. "She's a much better dancer overall. She's much better at musicality than I am. There are some songs I can't hear right. She can. So I count on her. Her body resonates with the music, so I can feel it through her. I depend on her, even though I'm supposed to be the lead. As dancers, you learn your partner's strengths and weaknesses and . . ."

"You deal with it," Cheri interjects. "We see couples screaming at each other off the floor. Or expressing their displeasure in other ways. We heard the woman of one top couple we were competing against say to her partner, 'When did you decide you didn't like our choreography?' It was very gentle, at least. He clearly had gone blank."

"We've learned to communicate in a way that we can move forward and progress, even if we have different skills," Art said. "In this case, Cheri is the better athlete. So I have to stuff my ego a bit and learn how to take coaching from my wife in a nice way. And she has to learn how to coach me the way I'm going to respond . . ."

"In a gentle way," Cheri responded. "We've gotten better at that."

Sharing the Joy

While dance clearly brings fulfillment to both couples, sometimes others can benefit as well. Scott and Bernie danced several years at the Wisconsin State Dance Championships. One year, the winning couple in their age group sought them out.

"We want to thank you," the couple said to Scott and Bernie. "When we came and watched you as a couple a few years ago, you were having so much fun. You looked like you were really into each other and having such a great time. That inspired us. We wouldn't have gotten serious about dance if we hadn't seen you out there and figured we could do it too."

"Wow—you never know how you influence people," Scott said, remembering the moment. "I never would have thought of us in that way."

From the Dance Pros and Researchers

So, how typical is this experience for other marital couples? There's been some limited research about how ballroom dancing impacts a marital relationship, and the results seem to affirm the Osborns' and the Rolnicks' experience.

In 2006, Ramona Hanke, a master's degree student in counseling psychology at the University of Pretoria in South Africa, used qualitative research methodology to follow three couples who danced at the local Arthur Murray Ballroom Dance Studios. Hanke selected three couples at random from the volunteers who stepped forward, did extensive interviews with them, and did not reveal their identities to the other dancers. Hanke herself had previously worked at an Arthur Murray studio.

Four different themes emerged from the research:

- The participating couples felt that ballroom dancing helped them improve their communication, making it more frequent and in-depth.

- They reported that their intimacy levels were enhanced, with more physical contact and more early-courtship feelings and emotions.
- The couples seemed to develop strategies for conflict management as they learned to dance.
- The couples recounted that while there were arguments along the way, they seemed to progressively make conscious decisions to use effective conflict-management strategies.

"Negotiation, investment, and cooperation appeared to be essential tools for the couples to succeed in dancing," Hanke concluded.

That's likely true. But I would add another essential tool: having a coach skilled in both dance and human nature.

Nathan Daniels, one of Art and Cheri's coaches, thinks of himself as a "marriage counselor" when he works with couples. His students tell me he's really good at it. When he became a ballroom dance judge years ago and could no longer compete with individual students, he focused on married couples, with marriages ranging from ten to nearly fifty years.

"I want them to be as good as they can be," Nathan said. "But it's more about managing them as a couple, making sure they always keep in mind that nobody is intentionally messing up. They seem to forget that."

Nathan understands that what's happening on the dance floor for a married couple isn't always about dance.

"Dance imitates life," he said. "You have to treat people well, and you have to watch your tone. After some forty-seven years of marriage, you would think you would know all your partner's buttons and that you wouldn't push them. But that doesn't happen. It's not necessary, and I don't tolerate it. It's like, 'No. You can't talk to others that way. I don't care who you are. It's just not conducive to anything, especially your relationship.' I tell them to stop it."

In Nathan's experience, gender doesn't distinguish. Men and women can be equally disrespectful and in need of redirection.

"It's just about validation," Nathan said. "If your partner says something, just listen! You are not perfect. *You* may be the one doing something wrong. So I just manage the couple to be lovely, kind human beings—*all* the time."

Yes, that's Nathan. Direct, no nonsense. That's what I love about him.

When Only One Partnership Remains

Of course, for some married couples, dance creates friction that builds over time and becomes too stressful for them. They choose to stop dancing for the sake of their relationship.

Sometimes there's tension because the partners have different goals and aren't on the same page as to what they wish to achieve. Other times, it's too much for them financially to pursue. Still other times, the couple needs to have separate interests because they already do too much together, or their priorities change and they decide to find other avenues to stay connected.

Life happens.

Perhaps the most painful scenario is when long-time spouses who are successful dance partners come to the difficult realization that they can no longer remain life partners. Usually, the dance partnership ends. But not always.

Next let's meet C. J. and Lorie Hurst.

Chapter 21

⌄

Can a Couple's Dance Passion Survive When Marriage Love Ends?

Remarkably, it can. Just ask C. J. and Lorie Hurst, my long-time neighbors in our downtown Minneapolis condominium. I've observed their relationship with my own eyes. Their authentic story moved me greatly and can be a bellwether for how other couples—dancers or not—might manage the dissolution of marriage.

As Lorie described, "I just thank the Lord. We started as friends and dance partners, and we're still friends and dance partners. In the middle, there was a marriage, and we've both decided we'll never regret it."

Lorie and C. J. met in group dance classes at a local studio in 2007. They were in their early thirties. Neither had danced before.

Though Lorie is a self-described tomboy, as a little girl she'd always had a "Cinderella dream" to learn to waltz because "it was so romantic and beautiful." She decided to try it when she received a dance studio coupon in a welcome packet as a new resident of Minneapolis.

Lorie attended classes and learned different dances nearly every night. It was a nice community for someone who didn't yet have friends in a new city. There were fewer gentlemen than ladies, so she was always happy to dance with "this geeky nerd with braces" who seemed friendly.

That was C. J. He may have looked like a nerd at first glance, but he was actually an athlete who was into sports and competitive volleyball. He'd started dance classes at the encouragement of a coworker. And yes, he'd seen the sensuous tango in the movie *Scent of a Woman.* C. J. found that "really cool." Meeting women would be a nice potential benefit.

C. J. was pretty shy about his ability to dance. "But I quickly realized that the worse you are, the less people watch you," he said. "As soon as I figured that out, I lost a lot of my inhibitions. Nobody's gonna be watching me anyway."

There were always more ladies than guys. So even though it took time for C. J. to learn new steps, he was enjoying himself and he felt appreciated. Before long, he realized that the people getting the most attention and best instruction were the ones taking private lessons and entering competitions.

"So I ended up entertaining the idea of competing fairly quickly," he said.

C. J. needed an amateur partner to compete. He approached Lorie at a dance party.

"Would you be my amateur partner?" he asked.

Lorie, distracted by her guest girlfriend, didn't know what "amateur partner" meant. But she gave him her phone number, to the surprise of her friend.

C. J. wasted no time in following up.

"He called under the pretense of getting together to practice, but he quickly started asking 'getting to know you' questions," recalled Lorie. "Then I realized he wanted more than just an amateur dance partner."

Shortly thereafter, C. J. signed them up for a dance competition. Lorie was surprised. She was terrified of competition; she just wanted to dance like Cinderella.

"What do you mean, going to a competition?" she asked him.

"You told me you would be my amateur dance partner," he said back.

That's when Lorie finally learned what "amateur partner" meant.

To make it even worse, C. J. had signed them up for dances within the first three levels of competition. Or so he thought. One of the three was the "novice" level. Despite its name, it's actually the fourth highest out of six. Now *that's* an ambitious start for a beginner couple who'd been dancing for only three months.

Lorie felt "tricked" into their first competition. "I found out later that C. J. doesn't communicate things. He takes the path of least resistance, and he just went ahead and signed me up. I think he thought it was easier to ask forgiveness than permission. So there we were. Oh God!"

"I did kind of drag Lorie into this," C. J. conceded. "I got very lucky that she was willing to give it a shot, even though I signed her up without her agreeing to it. I didn't explain 'amateur partner,' and I should have. And yes, I did sign us up for three levels."

The couple wound up winning one level at their first competition, and they even made callbacks at the higher novice level.

"We won all our 'newcomer' stuff," said C. J. "I've never seen Lorie bounce off the walls that high. It was an amazing thing. That was such a high, and it was so fun to experience that with her as a team. It felt like we were making strides and doing really well."

Of course, C. J. had competed all his life, including twenty years in volleyball. He was used to the highs, the adrenaline, the jitters, the winning.

Lorie was not. She'd never competed for anything athletic in her life. For her, the new experience was exhilarating. She was completely hooked. Sure, C. J. hadn't exactly been forthcoming with her at the outset. But it didn't take long for her to forgive him.

The couple kept taking lessons and entering competitions as they fell in love.

"We met dancing," Lorie said. "Dancing was a big part of our love story. I remember asking C. J. if we could please go on a date that wasn't a dance lesson, like a movie or a walk in a park. All he wanted to do was take dance lessons."

Dance, it seemed, was holding them together.

"We were on a good trajectory in dance," Lorie recalled. "And we got married in the middle of it."

The pastor who would be officiating their wedding insisted they do premarital counseling, and he counseled them to have a hobby together. They had trouble convincing the pastor that they were already constantly in each other's space with dance.

"The pastor made it sound like it was very important for our marriage that we do something together," Lorie said. "We were so proud of ourselves, that we were already doing that."

They married on January 29, 2011. They performed a waltz and rumba at their wedding.

"That was a big highlight for us," Lorie said. "Then we just hit the ground running and kept on dancing. Our marriage had high highs and many fun moments," she added, recalling their first few years. "We were fortunate to win most of our competitions. We just loaded up with medals and were full of adrenaline, hugging, and high-fiving each other."

But amid the highs were some lows.

"There were lots of challenges in our marriage too," Lorie said. "I was more romantic. I was so excited to be married to my dance partner that I tried to be a wife in our lessons, not just a dance partner. I would try to get flirty, but C. J. did not want any of that. I was supposed to turn off all that. C. J. looked at dance lessons as if we were athletes. It was convenient to be married to your dance partner, but it was supposed to be athletic."

C. J. acknowledged the same. "I had an awkward mind-set that I recognize now is not optimal. I certainly left a lot to be desired as a married dance partner. I should've been more relaxed about that. I was sometimes frustrated that lessons would get derailed with chitchat, which felt like a waste of money to me."

Over the next nine years, the couple entered three or four competitions each year, with instruction primarily from dance professional Paul Botes. They continued to grow into higher levels of competition, and they kept on winning. Their dance partnership kept growing stronger and stronger.

But their life partnership was not. Their marriage was falling apart.

When Life and Dance Partnerships No Longer Align

Lorie and C. J. made the painful decision to end their nine-year marriage in 2020. As Lorie explained, "We ended up being oil and water. We both said we married good people, but we were incompatible with our foundational pillars, such as religion, politics, communication, and intimacy. When it came to the things that hold a marriage together, we were on polar opposites. I think we went into it with stars in our eyes. Like the Beatles said, 'All you need is love.' We learned the hard way that oil and water are both fantastic things. But they didn't mix."

C. J. and Lorie quickly realized it was extremely difficult to keep their tensions from spilling over onto the dance floor.

"When a relationship falls apart, everything gets dragged through the dirt," Lorie said. "So our dance partnership got dragged through the dirt as well. There were some hurtful things said. I was made to feel I was a bad dance partner and that I wasn't giving enough. But I felt like I was giving everything I could."

When the marriage ended, so did their dance partnership. For Lorie, it was an overwhelming loss. She lost her husband, her home, her finances (C. J. was the breadwinner), and her dance. Making matters worse, it was 2020, and the COVID pandemic prevented Lorie from working in her profession as a massage therapist.

"I lost my whole life," she said.

As details of the divorce settlement were implemented, it became apparent that it was financially more practical for them to live in the same condominium building, but in two separate units. They wound up living several doors from each other, even though they'd tried geographically to go their separate ways.

"I'm not sure what God was thinking," Lorie said with a laugh.

C. J. had the financial resources to continue dancing. He began taking lessons with professional Natalie Botes. Lorie was missing dance deeply and felt starved without it. It was difficult to manage her feelings of wistfulness and jealousy. She did not seek another dance partner because in her mind, dance was always more than just an athletic pursuit; it was something romantic. It was her love story, and she couldn't fathom replacing C. J. with just an athletic partner.

That wasn't an issue for C. J. He went online immediately to find a new athletic dance partner. He auditioned three of them, working very hard to replace Lorie.

As time passed, Lorie and C. J. continued to run into each other in the hallway of their building, living just fifty feet apart. They began to rebuild a friendship and started to talk things through.

Lorie, who has strong faith, had been praying that some part of the relationship would be salvageable. "I knew I married a good person. I accepted the oil and water. I accepted the incompatibility. I just had a hard time accepting that we were completely walking away."

That didn't happen. Maybe because they found a way to walk together in that hallway.

"C. J. told me he learned a few things trying to find a replacement partner," Lorie said. "He said he learned how good I was, that I was better than he thought and not as easily replaceable as he thought. And one night he came to me."

"Lorie," he said, "would you be my amateur dance partner?"

It was the same question he'd asked fifteen years before.

Lorie didn't hesitate. "I burst into tears and threw my arms around him and said 'Yes!' about ten times."

Hearing this, I paused the joint interview of my good friends. I had to stop—my eyes were filled with tears. How much courage that took on both their parts!

"That was just fantastic," said C. J. as he told his side of the story. "I've been very, very thankful that she said yes again. I really wanted to dance with Lorie again, and I was excited to ask. But yes, there's a little humble pie there too. For certain. Lorie, as usual, was right about a number of things, and she's always very gracious about it."

Were there lessons learned for Lorie as well?

"Absolutely," she said. "C. J. says our dance partnership is working better now than before. I had to remove my romantic expectations. There's no flirting going on in our lessons anymore. I'm not insisting on bringing romance into it. It is an athletic pursuit, the way C. J. had wanted it. He lightened up a bit, and so did I, to meet in the middle. We have a partnership based on a solid friendship instead of a marriage. To return to our partnership, we decided we were going to be a lady and a gentleman, and we were going to treat each other with respect."

Lorie engaged in multiple Bible studies and group therapies after the divorce, eager to learn more about herself and her relationships. She applied those tools to the new partnership.

"I realized I was trying to pour love on C. J. But as a man, he probably needed respect. Things got harsh during the end of our marriage. We went back into our partnership thinking we both had to treat each other better. Both of us put respect at the forefront. We also felt gratitude that we could do this again. You combine gratitude with respect, and oh boy—we get a second chance! This is exciting! It's a good combination."

Lorie and C. J. are now dancing as partners into their fifties. They've risen through the ranks, competing at the fourth and fifth competition levels. Their goal remains the same: to compete successfully at the sixth level, called the championship level.

But aging has presented new challenges. Lorie's knee "popped" during the 2023 national competition, and she has been struggling with surgeries and therapies since. Knee replacements are likely in the future. And C. J. had to recover from a painful shoulder surgery.

But they continue to dance when physically able to do so—four to six lessons a week, as a couple or individually, with a professional.

"I don't think either of us wants to give up dancing for as long as humanly possible—as long as our bodies allow us," said C. J.

There is, of course, the question of how new romantic relationships with others would affect their dance partnership. That isn't currently an issue, though it may be someday.

"We're praying that other people would understand and still let us pursue a dance relationship," said Lorie. "But we don't take anything for granted. It's a real blessing to have what we have now. I hope it will last for a long time."

"It'll be challenging for us to get into other relationships because of the amount of time we spend working together," C. J. admitted. "And it's hard not to act like a couple. I just naturally fall into that with Lorie. It's so comfortable that way. Anyone looking at us will assume we are a couple."

There's one other factor that probably played a role in this inspiring story: Lorie's faith, which is fundamental in her life.

"I feel like what we're doing now is a reflection of the scriptures I grew up with, where God can take bad things and knit them together into something beautiful if we give him all the pieces. I've done a ton of praying. My faith was huge in helping me get over the divorce. I was a heap on the floor. I did the divorce-care program through a church, and it was so helpful."

Lorie's faith improved her own life and also her new partnership with C. J.

"I believe part of our success in the second chapter of our dance relationship is due to some emotional, mental, and spiritual growth. I have to credit my faith for a lot of that growth. I have to credit God with helping me heal, helping me change, helping me grow, and blessing our efforts. I was working on me. My goal was to become a better person. That also means a better dance partner. That also means a better friend."

Yes, they started as friends and dance partners, and they are still friends and dance partners. In the middle, there was a marriage.

"It didn't last," Lorie said. "But it was a beautiful chapter, and it's left us where we are today. We're so enjoying each other for what we can give each other, without worrying about what we couldn't give each other."

C. J. nodded. "Lorie has a beautiful way with words. She also has a great perspective. It was wonderful to start dancing with Lorie again. We're still excited about learning and getting better. I think we're having more fun in our lessons than before. I've certainly grown and learned to lighten up and have more fun, which was desperately needed, I'm sure. It was eye opening to recognize just how much easier it was to dance with Lorie than anybody else."

Yes, things can be salvaged and second chances given. Beautiful things can come from the darkest moments as we all dance through life.

Chapter 22

Family Resilience Through Generations

The dance community is making room for young people and their families. More and more dance showcases and competitions include sessions featuring students ranging from pre-school to high school to be critiqued by judges. In Minnesota, dozens of young people dominate the dance floor in these sessions, particularly in the International Ballroom and Latin styles. Nearly all the students come from the Dance with Us America studio, and they dance under the watchful eyes of their teachers and studio owners, Gene and Elena Bersten.

This is a vivid illustration of Gene and Elena's remarkable legacy. They have taught hundreds of kids over twenty years in Minnesota. Both started teaching at the tender age of fifteen; Elena taught in Russia before coming here.

Their students experience success on and off the dance floor. The studio has produced fifteen national champions, including members of the Bersten family. One student taught ballroom dance to his fellow midshipmen before he graduated from the US Naval Academy.

Today, the Berstens teach students of all ages, while they themselves compete professionally in their American Rhythm partnership, having become national professional champions and world finalists.

"Children can learn dance at four years old," explained Elena. "It makes their memory better and their movements better. They become more confident than other children."

Gene and Elena's own daughters are proof positive. In 2025, at just age twelve, Isabella was dancing ten dances and competing at the advanced Open level in International Latin and Ballroom. Gabriella, three years younger, was competing at the Silver and Gold levels in the same styles. And even six-year-old Nika is already competing at the Bronze level.

Their family dance story does not come by accident. Both Gene and Elena come from families immersed in dance. Their teaching mirrors the Russian cultural teaching they experienced from their own dance coaches. Gene's and Elena's journeys were not always easy. But throughout it all, they were driven by unwavering commitment to work hard, set goals, and achieve results.

"We didn't have anything special," recalled Gene of his years growing up. "It was just that 'drive.' Anyone can achieve anything if you really want to. You really have to *want* to. If you look at the success story of anyone who achieves anything, they all had one thing in common—they all had that drive, and they all wanted it more than the other person. Whoever wants it more is going to achieve it."

Gene's family instilled that ethos in him. When Gene's parents moved to the United States, they had to give up their citizenship in Belarus. Gene's mom was an engineer; his dad a recent army veteran. As Gene explains, they moved to their new country with "literally no money in their pocket." They didn't speak a word of English.

"My parents are some of the hardest workers you'll ever meet," Gene said. "That's where I got my work ethic."

Gene's parents became US citizens. His dad started fixing cars and is a mechanic today. His mom, Raisa Bersten, cleaned houses while she went back to school, working her way into new careers. She is currently manager of neurosurgery at Children's Hospitals and Clinics of Minnesota.

Gene started dancing ballroom, ballet, and jazz at around eleven years old. His first instructor was Robert Foster, who made dancing a "big part" of Gene's life. Gene and his sister Melanie (five years younger) and brother Alan (six years younger) were "all into it."

Then Gene's mom and a partner started a studio in Minnesota. At age fifteen, Gene started training with world finalist Aleksandra Gisher, who has been his coach for sixteen years since. Gene's parents didn't have money for all three kids to take lessons, so Gene received the majority of the coaching and then would teach Melanie and Alan.

"We spent every free minute at the studio dancing," said Gene.

The Berstens would arrange for Aleksandra to come to Minnesota every two weeks. "That was very expensive," Gene said. "She lived with us and was like a mother figure to us. She guided our dance careers, taught us how to practice and how not to waste our time with it."

Not having a local instructor posed some challenges, but it also provided some unexpected benefits.

"When people have their coaches with them every day, they take it for granted," Gene explained. "We didn't have that. We had to soak up everything while coaches were here because we knew when they left, we were on our own. We tried to get the most out of that and then afterwards work every day."

By age sixteen, Gene's routine was set: He'd pick up his dance partner from school, practice a few hours, teach lessons, and then, at the end of the day, practice some more.

"What helped us to be better is that we were teaching at the same time," Gene said. "I was teaching mainly kids. We had a huge kids' program here in Minnesota when we started. It was mainly the Russian community who came to support us."

One of Gene's students was his brother, Alan, as we learned in Chapter 19.

"My brother and I were very competitive," Gene said. "I taught him four to six times a week. Family teaching family is the hardest thing to do. Every lesson was very personal because of our competitiveness. But whatever I said to him was because I always wanted him to be better."

Gene helped both his siblings adopt an "If we want to win, we first have to win in our heads" approach. It seemed to work. All three Berstens—Gene, Melanie, and Alan—became national Latin champions in the junior and youth divisions and went on to become dance teachers.

Building self-confidence can also have its downside, though.

"People used to say when I was younger that I was cocky and arrogant," Gene admitted. "But it was taught to me—my coaches taught me that. Before dance, I was really self-conscious. I didn't speak very good English. My parents didn't have a lot of money. And I didn't have nice clothes. In dance, they taught me the opposite—to be confident and happy in what I do. We were brought up like this, to learn to have such high self-worth."

Meanwhile, thousands of miles away, Elena's family in Orel, Russia, was also deeply immersed in dance. Elena's mom is a dance teacher, judge, competition organizer, and studio owner in Russia.

Though her mom wanted eight-year-old Elena to start dancing in the studio, Elena would have none of it.

"They put a good boy partner with me," she said. "I was so shy. I didn't want to dance with a boy. I said I wouldn't go anymore. Mom tried again, and I said no."

So Elena's mom put her into gymnastics instead. Then when Elena was twelve, her mom enticed her to dance in a roundabout way.

"Mom offered to teach dance for free to my classmates at school. The principal agreed. That was fun for us. Later, students could sign up for more lessons at the studio. And that is how I started to dance."

Now that is a clever mom!

Elena attended intense dance camps in Moscow, then returned to Orel to teach and become a judge. Later, she created a dance show based in Moscow, performing before royalty and celebrities.

"To live in Moscow was hard and very expensive," Elena said. "But I got good experience with the dance show, so I went back and forth between Moscow and Orel."

Elena sent her dance videos to several agencies. One recruited her for Burn the Floor, a prestigious international dance troupe that traveled around the world. It was a great career move—with benefits.

That's how she met Gene in Florida in 2008. They worked together every day yet somehow found free time to be together. They toured globally and continued their long-distance relationship after the tour.

Elena began teaching in the Bersten family studio when she visited Minnesota. "We fell in love," she recalled. "We understood we couldn't live without each other."

They prepared immigration documents for Elena to move to Minnesota in 2011. They got engaged on the Eiffel Tower in Paris and married in Minnesota on September 4, 2011. Elena became a US citizen in 2016.

"We're very compatible," Gene said. "We're like best friends, together 24/7. That would drive some people nuts. We enjoy it."

Dance continued as the family's central focus. Both Gene and Alan auditioned for Season 10 of the television series *So You Think You Can Dance*. Both passed all auditions.

"It came down to me and Alan, and they took the younger cast that year," Gene recalled. "The oldest dancer was eighteen or nineteen, and I was about twenty-five. Alan eventually placed in the top six. They invited me for the next season, but I said no because we then had a child."

Alan later performed with Burn the Floor, then joined the dance troupe of the hit television show *Dancing with the Stars*. He soon became a dance professional matched with celebrity dancers. He and partner Bachelorette Hannah Brown won the

Season 28 championship in 2019. Then in November 2024, Alan and his partner, Ilona Maher, an Olympic rugby bronze medalist, were the runner-up champions.

"Alan and I are very close," Gene continued. "He's still my best friend. We talk every day on the phone about everything. I always say I'm his biggest critic and his biggest fan. I 'feel' how he dances. We feel for each other. It's more stressful watching him dance than dancing myself. Even now on *Dancing with the Stars*, I look at all his routines before he dances them."

Gene feels the same thing when he competes with his students.

"I'm more nervous for their results than I am for my own. I want them to do well. They work so hard, and I think they deserve it. I always want my students to dance 150 percent, so after they're done, they're not thinking to themselves, 'I wish I had done more.'"

So, what are Gene and Elena's dreams for the future?

"My main thing in life is always a happy, healthy family," Gene said. "That's number one. I want my kids to be successful in anything they do. That's what I tell all parents whose kids take lessons here," he added. "If they want their kids to be good at anything, they have to go 100 percent. You can't do anything halfway. If parents don't encourage their children to work more, they're not going to do it. I don't know any kid who wants to sit in the studio for hours and work his butt off. But anyone good at anything works their butt off. That's the difference between growing up in America and in other countries. It's a difference in culture."

For the Bersten daughters, it's even more than 100 percent.

"I expect more from them than other kids," Gene said. "But they deliver. It's tough love. If I didn't think they were capable, I wouldn't push. I start them the right way right away. I teach them hard work. Of course, we want them to have fun, too, and they do. But they have to work."

Elena agreed. "When they're four years old, we push them a little more here in the studio. We can ask more of them. They have lots of lessons with us and different instructors and partners."

With babies and a studio, the couple chose to delay their own desire to dance together competitively until 2021. After training less than two years, they became the 2022 US National Professional Rising Star champions in American Rhythm. In 2023 and 2024, they became World Professional Rhythm finalists. In 2025, at ages thirty-seven (Gene) and forty-one (Elena), they aspire to place in the top three. Both are certified national judges.

All this as they raise a young family in life and dance.

"When we practice, we are very efficient," Gene said. "Because I don't know any pros at this level who have three kids. It's hard to sustain this level."

Gene and Elena also want to build a community of dance.

"We want to leave the next generation of dancers better off than we were," Gene said. "We want to grow this. We want to have lots of Dance with Us America studios. We have brought over new instructors from Russia."

As part of their mission to grow a dance community, the three Berstens—Gene, Elena, and Alan—combined forces in 2023 to buy the successful Snow Ball DanceSport Competition, located in a suburb of Minneapolis. They are successfully continuing this legacy event that was originally cofounded and ably organized for twenty years by dance professional Donna Edelstein.

Today, the Berstens continue to teach students in all International and American dance styles. They acknowledge that their strict technical focus and high expectations aren't a fit for every student.

But their mission and life experience will inspire anyone.

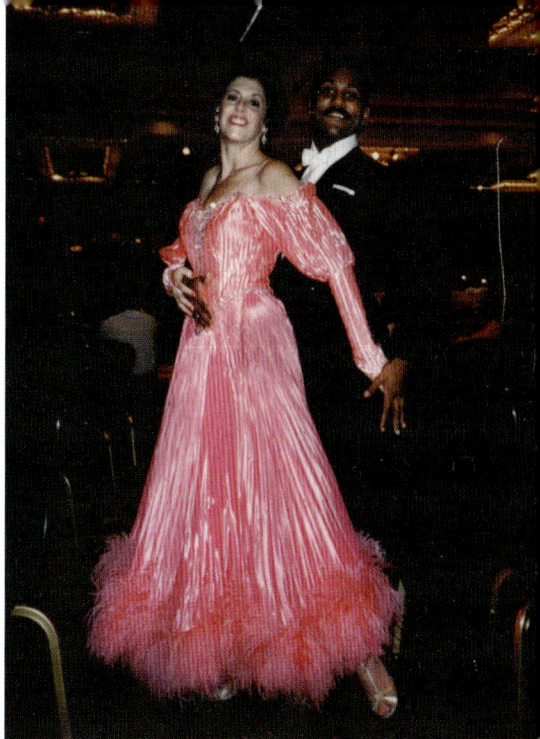

Ember with instructor
Nathan Daniels at competition
around 1991 (Chapter 18)

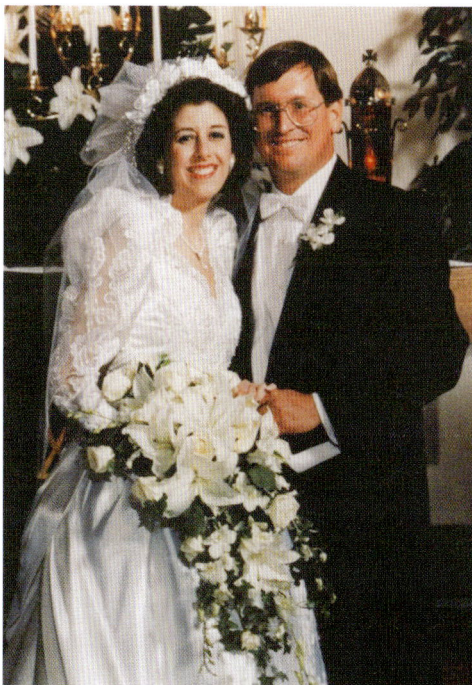

Ember marries Michael
Junge in 1993, who
doesn't dance a step.
(Chapter 18)

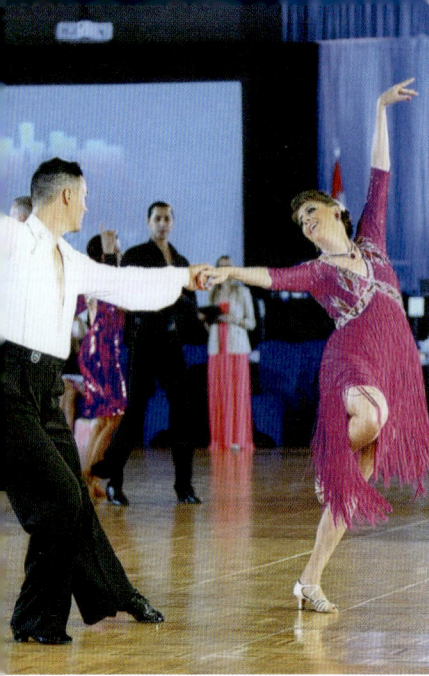
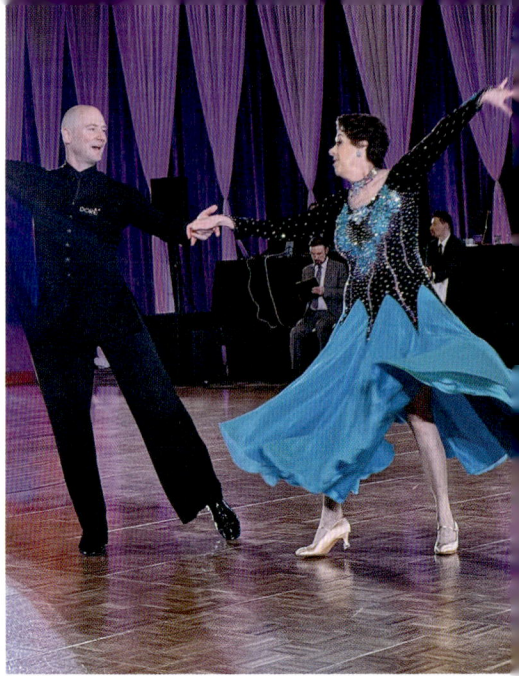
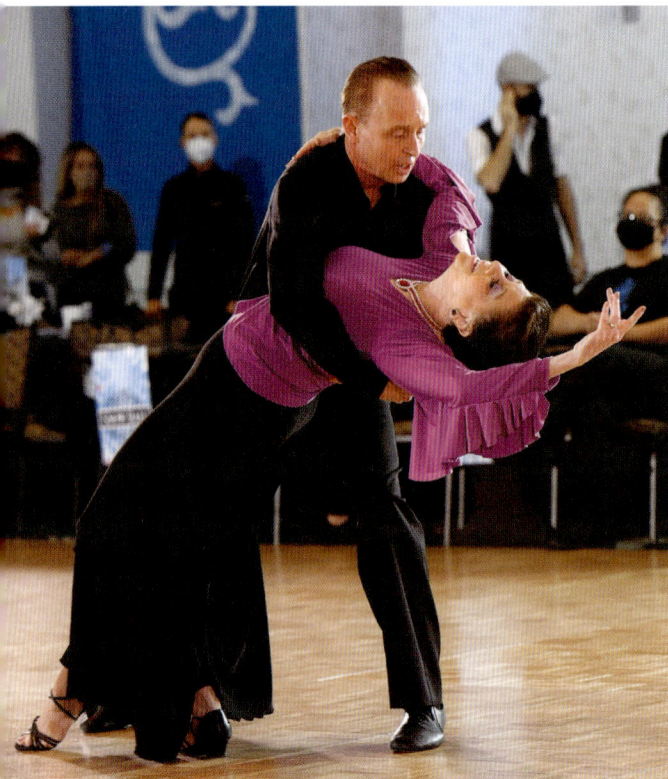

Competition nerves: with instructors Gordon Bratt (top left), Martin Pickering (top right), and Scott Anderson (bottom) (Chapter 19)

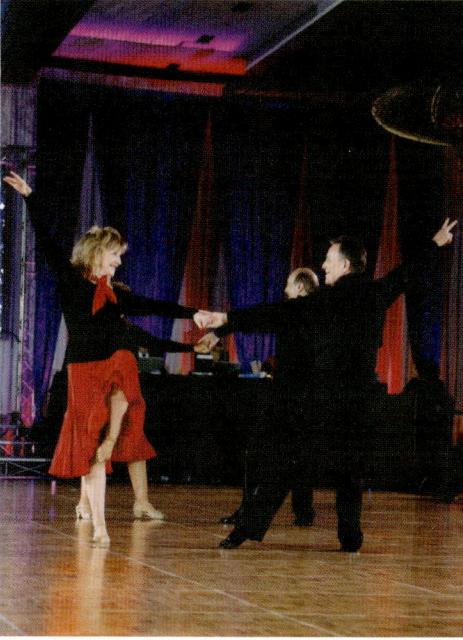

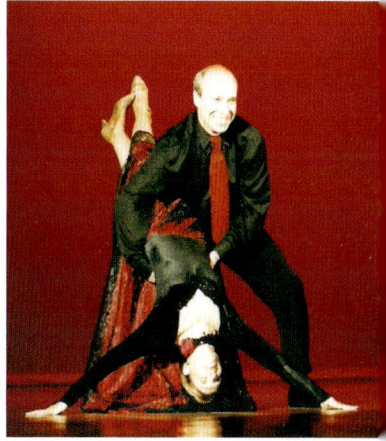

Mid-life Tango! Dance formation teammates Scott and Bernie Osborn (left) and Art and Cheri Rolnick. (Chapter 20)

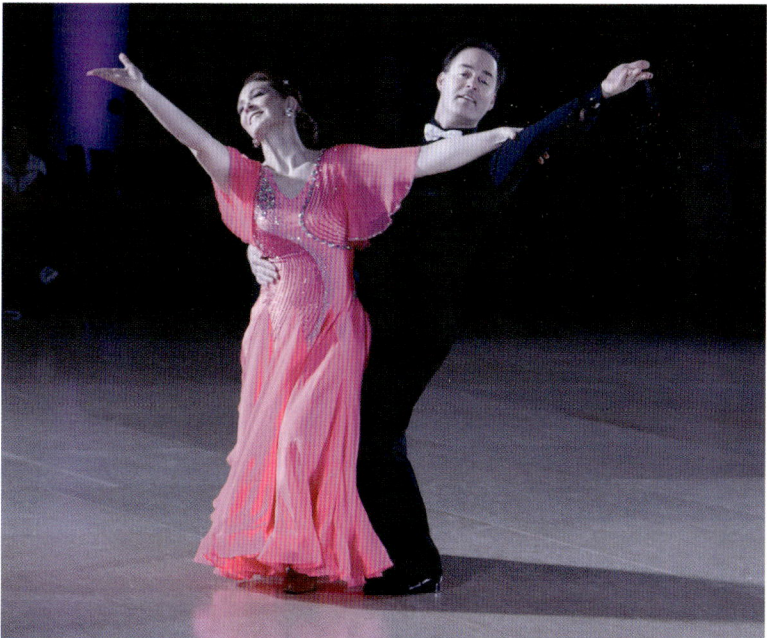

C. J. and Lorie Hurst: dance partners for life (Chapter 21)

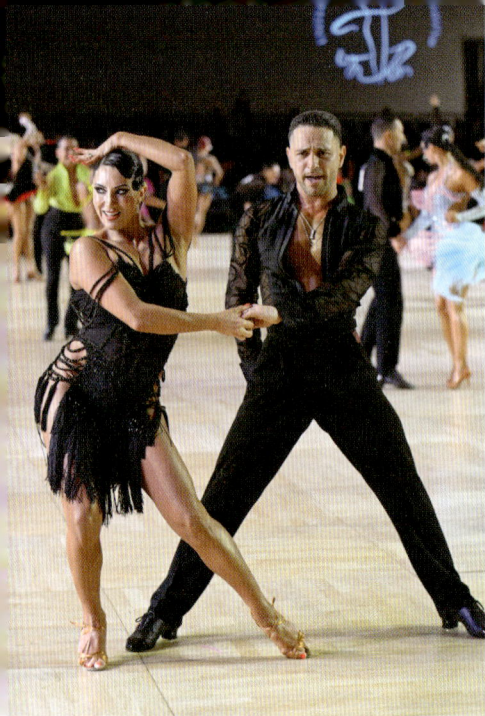

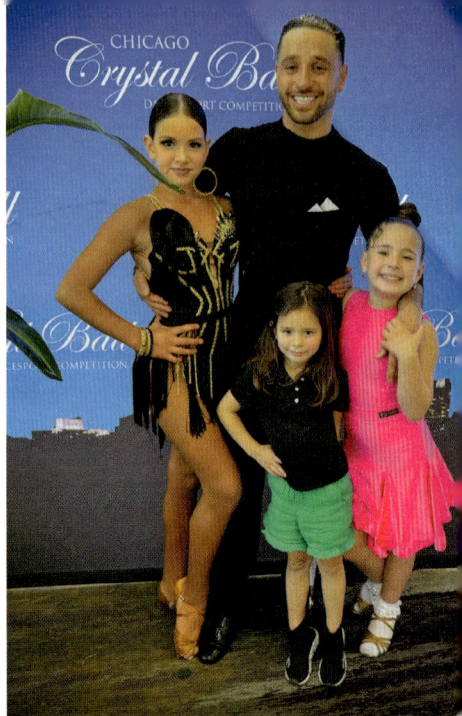

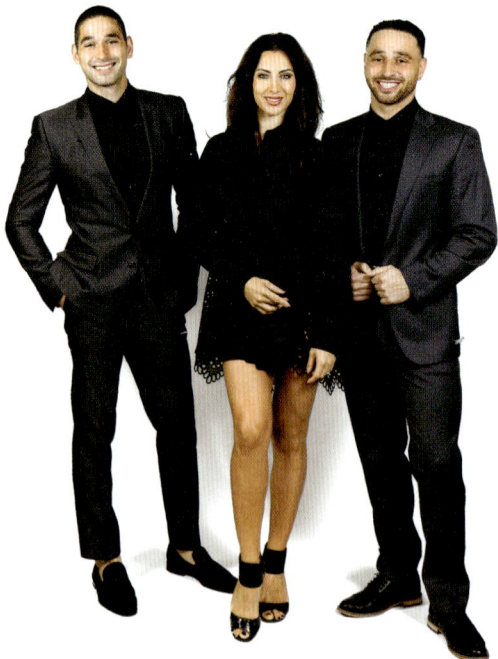

All in the Bersten family:
Gene, Elena, Isabella, Nika,
and Gabriella. Brother Alan
(left of trio). (Chapter 22)

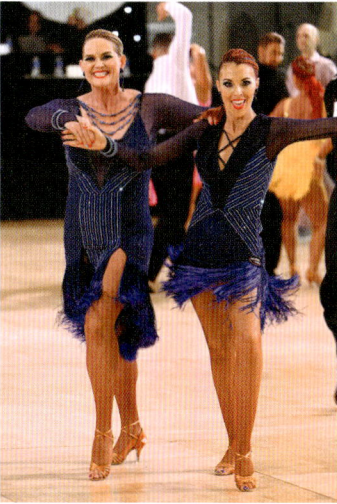

"The Girls in Blue"—instructor
Heather Wudstrack (right) and
Sarah Merz (Chapter 23)

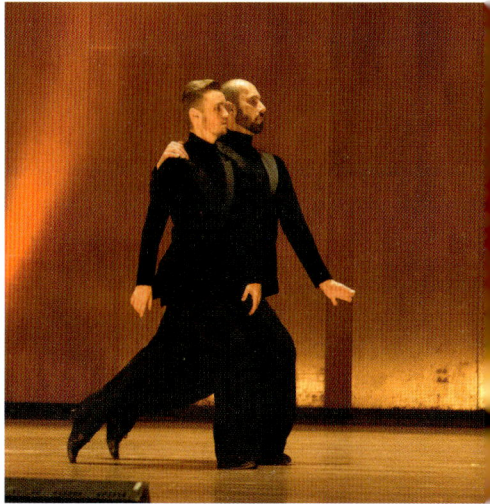

Professional partners Alex and Kato
(Chapter 23)

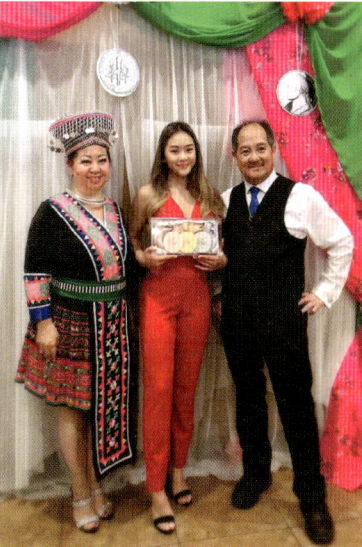

Two Hmong women break barriers:
Olympic Gold Medalist Suni Lee and
clan grandparents Cheu and Choua Lee
(Choua is first Hmong elected official
in nation). (Chapter 24)

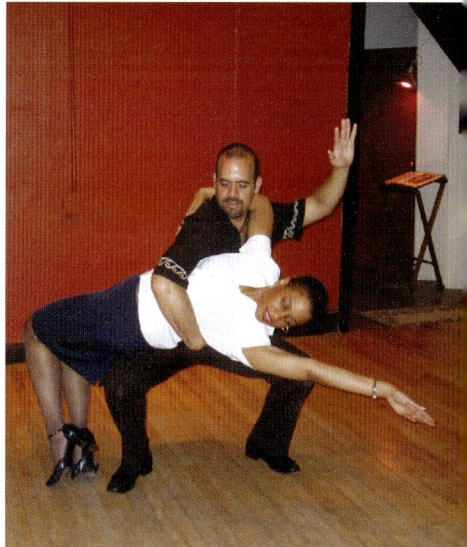

Psychologist Dr. Don DeBoer: talk therapy by day,
Salsa "therapy" by night (Chapter 25)

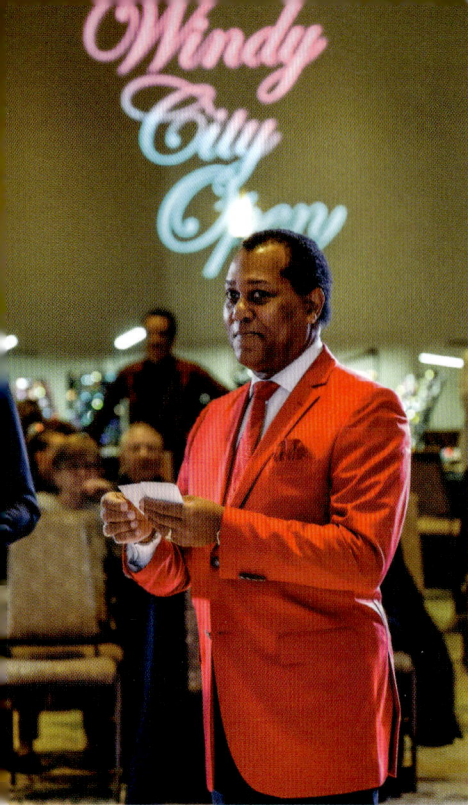

Nathan Daniels, ballroom dance judge
(Chapter 26)

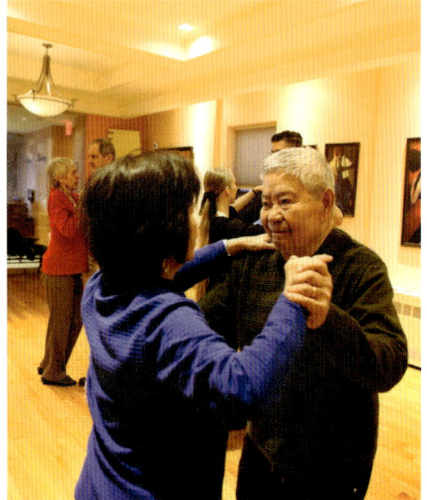

People with dementia dance in class in
New York City. (Chapter 28)

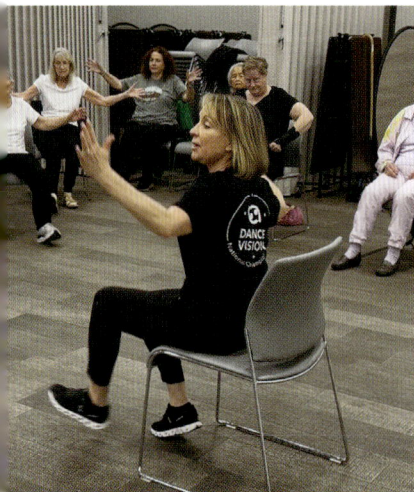

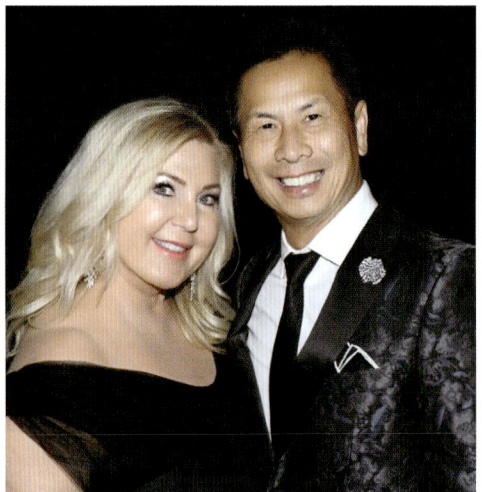

Dance Vision Foundation founders Wayne and Donna Eng (right) count on dance professional
Maria Hansen (left) to bring dance to those living with dementia. (Chapter 28)

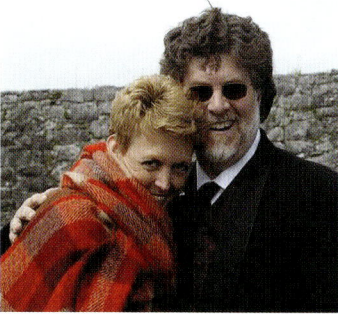

Ballet teacher Linda Muir helps husband Michael Finney to reduce his Parkinson's impairment. (Chapter 29)

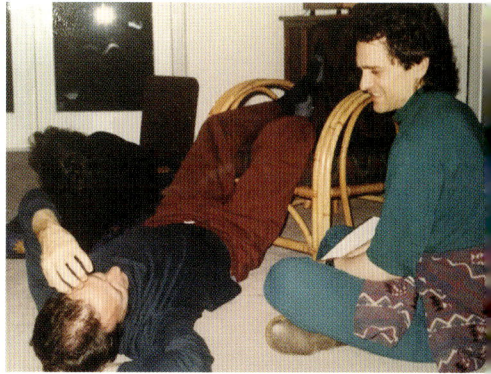

Dance/Movement Therapist Michael Gardos Reid (right) consults with a colleague. (Chapter 32)

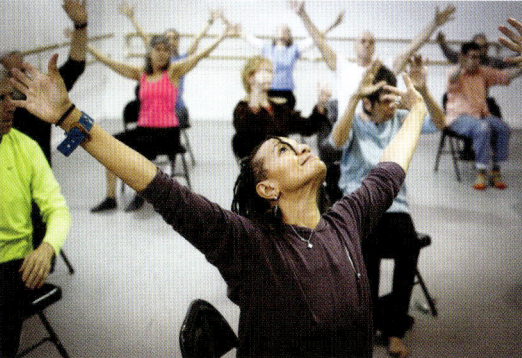

Globally, Dance for PD® classes are in 450 sites and growing. (Chapter 30)

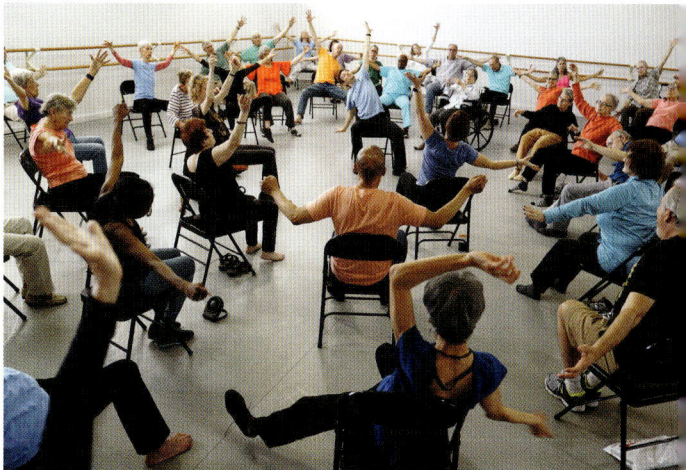

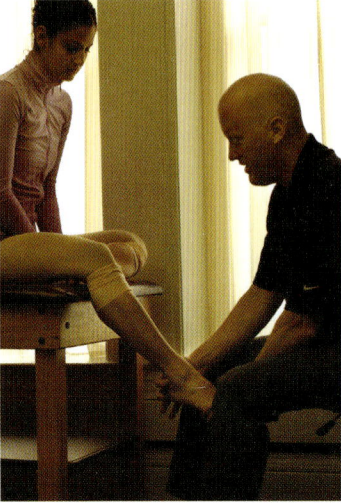

Dr. Brad Moser: the "Go-To" physician
for Dance Medicine in Minnesota
(Chapter 33)

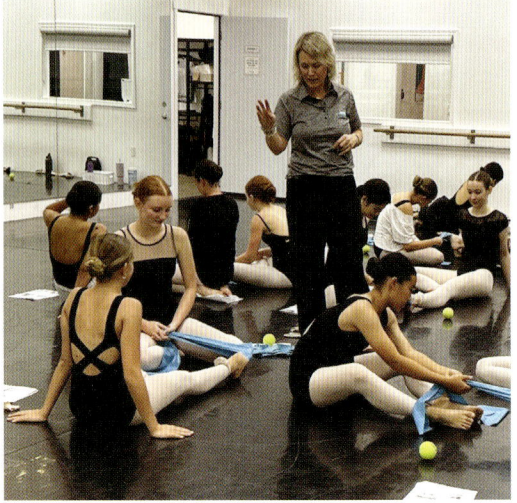

Dr. Megin Sabo John, a physical therapist and dancer,
specializes in dance medicine. (Chapter 33)

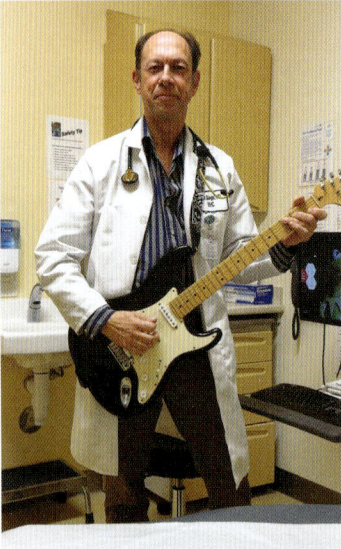

Physician and musician Dr. Alan Siegel,
cofounder of Social Prescribing USA
(Chapter 35)

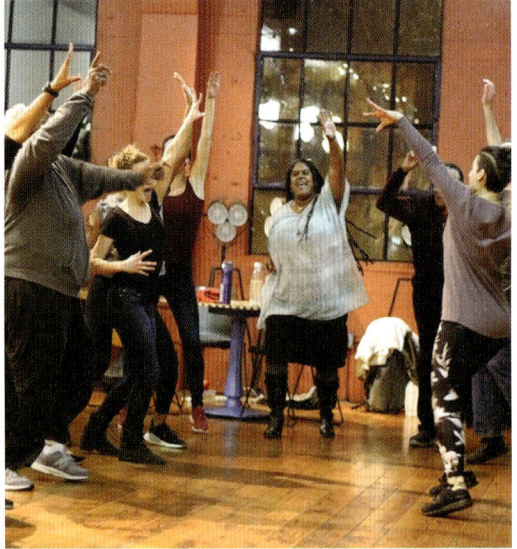

A "Community as Medicine" session
in full action! (Chapter 36)

PART IV

Breaking through Gender, Racial, and Cultural Barriers

The ballroom dance world has traditionally been conservative in nature, populated primarily by white individuals with discretionary financial resources. Gratefully, that is changing, for the benefit of dancers and the community.

Resilient individuals of different cultures, colors, and gender identities and orientations are breaking through the ballroom world, overcoming barriers, and opening doors for others.

Chapter 23

⌄

Same-Sex Dance Breaks Through Ballroom Dance World

Picture two dancers in beautiful partnership, dancing a lovely waltz or feisty cha-cha. Your picture no doubt includes a gentleman gently leading his lady follower.

The sight of two gentlemen waltzing together in matching tuxes probably doesn't come to mind. Nor does the sight of two women dancing together in their body-fitting Latin dresses. Why? Because it just didn't happen in the traditional ballroom dance world.

Until now.

Today, same-sex couples dance together in ballroom studios around the country. The reasons for same-sex dance are as varied as the dancers.

Why such partnerships? Some same-sex spouses and life partners enjoy dancing together. Some people feel safer dancing with a person of the same gender. Some mothers wish to take lessons with their daughters. Some people pair with dance partners of the same gender for educational purposes because learning the role traditionally danced by the opposite gender helps them become better competitors or teachers. Some students can't find quality instructors of the opposite gender in their geographic area. And some women dance instructors struggle to find enough male students to support a lifestyle in the profession they love.

Yes, the doors of the traditional ballroom dance world officially opened in fall of 2019, when the National Dance Council of America (NDCA) changed its long-standing rule defining a "couple" to allow same-sex couples to participate in accredited dance competitions. The NDCA oversees and regulates the most traditional, or mainstream, circuit of ballroom dance competitions in the United States. There are dozens of NDCA competitions, and the rule change applied to all levels of partnership: partnerships between two professional dancers, partnerships between professional teachers and amateur students (pro-am), and partnerships between two amateur dancers.

The rule change was a big deal, though it was anything but easy. The legal struggle took two full years. And though the rules have changed, some hearts and minds still have not. Change takes time. Those leading change—especially cultural change—must demonstrate and sustain a personal and political resilience few of us will ever experience.

Three same-sex dance couples broke through ballroom barriers and helped pave the way for others. Their impact still resonates nationally, with every competition they attend. And their followers grow every year. They are proof positive that resilience generates results.

Alex and Kato: Personal Transition and Industry Transformation

When the rule change for same-sex dancing occurred on September 23, 2019, Alex and Kato were spouses and retired champion professional dance partners.

For Alex Tecza, grounded in science as a microbiologist, the rule change allowed a "scientific experiment" where he could "create a different form of ballroom dancing born out of the original that could coexist alongside the traditional form." For Kato Lindholm, who had transitioned from female Katja to male Kato in 2017, the rule change gave people "the freedom to be who they are, dance what they want, with whomever they want."

As you read this, you might jump to the conclusion that Alex and Kato spearheaded the NDCA's rule change, but that's not the case. The couple was never directly involved in the legal fight for the rule change. For that matter, the legal fight traces back prior to Kato's transition, before they even were the same gender.

Rather, the fight traces back to when Alex broke his foot and Carol Lockwood, their long-time dance student, took a fateful step in her personal dance journey. How this all played out is an incredible—and resilient—story.

But let's start at its beginning.

Alex started dancing in Poland in 1989, when his entire high school class joined a ballroom dance club. His competitive nature in sports emerged immediately. When his family came to America about a year and a half later, he sought dance opportunities near his home, taking classes at the University of Illinois at Urbana-Champaign (UIUC) as well as taking lessons from a ballroom dance coach in Chicago.

Alex and his dance partner, a fellow UIUC student, competed together, rising to amateur national finalists in International Ballroom. When they ended their amateur partnership in 2001, Alex placed an ad on a global dance website to search for a new high-level partner to pursue his serious competition goals.

Meanwhile, Katja, who "was born into dance," grew up in Denmark. Her parents were professional dancers and teachers with a home studio. Around age twenty, Katja began competing in Sweden with a Swedish dance partner, and they won multiple Swedish national championships.

Eventually, Katja experienced burnout and a subsequent failed dance partnership, so she took some time to recover. Shortly thereafter, she answered Alex's ad. With background checks from coaches and email exchanges with Alex about their mutual level of commitment, Katja decided to travel to the United States in 2003. She intended it to be a three-month tryout with Alex—but she never really left. The partnership clicked on and off the dance floor.

The couple married in 2003, turned professional in 2004, and opened a studio in 2005. They did well in International Ballroom style in US competitions. All was good.

Then one day, Carol Lockwood asked if Alex and Katja could instruct her in the American Smooth style of dance. The request wasn't unusual. As the name suggests, American Smooth is an American style of dance, while International Ballroom is European. American students prefer American Smooth when learning waltz, foxtrot, and tango. American Smooth allows more freedom and expression in movement since partners are not always connected in full-body contact.

Neither Alex nor Katja knew anything about American Smooth. They had to learn it from scratch. "We discovered American Smooth in early 2007 as kind of comic relief, and to find joy in dance again," recalled Alex.

And did they ever find joy! Their technical International Ballroom training shone through in their American Smooth dancing, and they made "an incredible leap in ranks." Soon they chose to focus solely on American Smooth. They placed in the finals at major competitions across the country, and they won the Professional Rising Star category at the Ohio Star Ball competition.

Then in 2010, they retired from competitions. With their highly accomplished professional career now behind them, they concentrated on teaching and developing their own style of ballroom.

Time passed, and 2017 turned out to be the most pivotal year in their lives. They began thinking about closing their professional studio. At the time same, Katja was "sorting out things inside" and making the decision to transition to Kato, a male.

His decision seemed to provide another reason for closing the studio. The couple worried about the public reaction to a same-sex couple operating a dance studio.

"That is not a good business strategy—I can tell you that," Kato said.

"Let's be honest," Alex added. "Ballroom dancing is a rather conservative form of business—at least it was at the time. So I didn't want to risk having a big studio and no students because of the transition." Indeed, the couple lost about 50 percent of their students after Kato's transition.

While this was unfolding in Alex and Kato's life, something bigger and more impactful was unfolding as well. Prior to 2017 and Kato's transition, Alex had broken his foot. This prompted Carol to take lessons with Katja as her instructor. Since they were the same gender, the women needed to decide who would lead and who would follow. Carol chose to lead, with Katja following. Carol liked the leader role, so she continued with it even when Alex's foot was healed and he returned as her instructor.

Carol and Alex decided to compete under this reversed-role arrangement when they discovered a loophole in the NDCA rules: While a "couple" was clearly defined as a man and a woman, the rules didn't specify which role each needed to play. So for two competitions, Carol led and Alex followed.

It didn't take long for the NDCA to react. That same year, the regulatory body clarified the rule to define a "couple" as a man as leader and a woman as follower. Ironically, Carol had caused the rule to become even more conservative.

"She was really ticked off," Alex said.

Carol, a lawyer, started legal proceedings to change the rules to allow same-sex couples to dance together in competitions and to allow mixed couples to reverse roles. The complex battle took over two years.

Though Alex and Kato were not directly involved in Carol's crusade, they knew they could play an important role—and not just as Carol's instructors and supporters. Alex and Kato decided that if the rule changed, they would come out of retirement and enter an NDCA competition as a professional same-sex couple. They'd *have* to, they realized. If a highly reputed, formerly male-female couple could make a comeback as a male-male couple, then Carol's fight would be even more worthwhile.

"We wanted to show that this rule change can have much larger impact for other partnerships, not just one particular case," Alex said.

In anticipation of the rule change, Alex and Kato prepared new routines in American Smooth and, for the first time, in American Rhythm. To gain experience, they entered a North American Same-Sex Partner Dance Association (NASSPDA) competition in January 2019. The NASSPDA is a much smaller, nontraditional competition circuit compared to the NDCA. Alex and Kato won the NASSPDA national championships in both styles.

"This was our return from retirement," Alex said. "A big comeback as a same-sex couple."

Alex and Kato were breaking traditions in other ways as well. They chose to role-switch multiple times during each routine. That meant that during the same dance, sometimes Alex would lead and other times Kato would.

"We build choreography so we can switch seamlessly within a dance," Alex explained. "You may start as a lead, and in five seconds, you become a follow. And by the time people realize you are a follow, you are back leading again. The whole point is to make it look like you can't even see the switch. That's what I would say was our biggest contribution—there are no assigned roles."

While Alex and Kato don't claim to have come up with the role-switching concept, they did get people's attention when they did it.

Later that year, in September 2019, the NDCA rule change finally came through. Carol's crusade had been a success.

The Chicago Harvest Moon Ball Dancesport Championship, which is part of the mainstream NDCA circuit, was just two weeks later. Alex and Kato were ready to make their NDCA debut as a same-sex professional couple.

For their American Smooth routine, they wore matching tuxedos. They surprised many when they made the finals from a semifinal round and then placed seventh overall in all dances. That's pretty remarkable in the traditional ballroom world.

"We were in a position where we could make an impact based on our previous results," Kato said. "We had achieved something. We were known in the dance world amongst the judges. When we showed up, the judges had to decide what to do. The fact it was us maybe had a bit more power than if some newcomers had done it. We might have helped the cause a little more."

Alex and Kato entered one more competition, but then the pandemic started in 2020. At that point, they chose to retire (for good) from competition as a professional couple.

So, was the long and difficult journey to the rule change worth it, for them personally as well as for others in the ballroom world? Both Alex and Kato gave a resounding yes—but for different reasons.

For Kato, it was important on a very personal level. "As much as I had always loved dancing and had seen myself as a dancer growing up, I'd always felt there wasn't necessarily a natural space for me in dancing. I had to bend over backwards sometimes to fit into what was expected. My experience of dancing after transition is completely different. I'm very free. I feel great about it. I feel completely at home in dancing and in myself. Personally, it means a lot."

He paused before continuing.

"On a broader level, I can only imagine other people having the same feelings as I had. There will be some out there who would like to be more free in their dancing. That's what this rule change really was. It gives people the freedom to be who they are, dance what they want, with whomever they want. I think it has great positive implications for everybody."

With his scientific, analytical mind, Alex saw the rule change in a unique way. "It was like an intellectual experiment experience," he said. "It was very educational because up to that time, dance was very gender based."

He noted how, previously, judges might have scored a mixed couple well because the woman was "feminine in her movements" or because the man "strong." But after the rule change, such notions wouldn't work—especially not for Alex and Kato.

"To me, we had to create a different form of ballroom dancing that was born out of the original that can coexist alongside the traditional form," he said. "I've heard from others that we've had an impact on them. It was not a decision for us to do it to have an impact, but it did. And we are happy we can inspire some people, even though we might not necessarily be active [as a professional couple] right now."

So, where *are* they now, five years after the rule change? Both Alex and Kato continue to teach dance and compete in pro-am competitions with their students.

Alex, now fifty-two, teaches credit courses in the dance department at the University of Illinois. His syllabus includes teaching all students how to lead and follow, regardless of gender. He also teaches privately at rented spaces and in local fitness centers and hospitals. His goal is to make dance his primary career, but he always has microbiology to fall back on.

He is currently working on his master's in fine arts at UIUC, where he will soon present his written and oral thesis and choreographed presentation. His thesis is about the intersection of art and science, with a specific focus on partnering and how it relates to atomic interactions of molecules.

(Huh? Whatever works!)

Kato, now forty-seven, teaches part-time, including teaching the collegiate dance team at UIUC. He's been doing that for fifteen years, focusing on teaching nongendered roles, where everyone learns to lead and follow. Kato enjoys building the next generation of dancers in the collegiate competition circuit, which has historically been more liberal.

"In collegiate competitions," Kato said, "dancers can mix and match as they see fit for partnerships. A girl can lead. A guy can follow. Same-sex couples can dance. Under the rules, they just can't do role-switching during the dances. But we can stay true to our beliefs in the confines of the rules."

Kato's full-time job is as head cheesemaker at a local farmstead, where he's spent the last three years learning to make cheese.

"Everything you learn in dancing is relevant to cheesemaking," Kato said. "You've got to pay attention to detail, got to have good timing, and you have to be willing to clean up your shit!" he added with a laugh.

This year, Kato was awarded first place in three categories in the American Cheese Society's North American championship.

"It's the best North American cheese," Alex said proudly. "It's like the US Dance Championships in cheesemaking!"

And five years later, how has same-sex dance been accepted in the competitive ballroom dance world?

"I think it's getting more and more accepted," Kato replied. "But there will always be people who prefer the conservative way. That's just how it is. When we first came out dancing same-sex, people were like '*What*? This is weird! I don't know what to do with this.' Now it's 'Oh, there's a same-sex couple.' I feel, at least from other competitors, that there's been a lot of support, a lot of, 'This is cool. I wish I could do that.' And I say to them, 'But you can. You can do it. You don't have to be special to do it. And it doesn't have to have anything to do with your gender identity or sexuality. Everyone can do it.'"

Heather and Sarah: Showcasing Their Female Power

Sarah Merz was enjoying her beginning ballroom dance journey with several male instructors at a studio in central Wisconsin, near Wausau. During that time, she became good friends with professional teacher Heather Wudstrack at the studio. They bonded in part because Heather instructed Sarah's son Luke, who was just twelve years old when he started taking lessons.

Then the pandemic came. The ballroom studio permanently closed. The male instructors chose to retire. Sarah's lessons ended.

Heather, a twelve-year veteran teacher, reached out to her students to assess their interest in returning to dance if she started a studio of her own. Many said yes. So she moved down the street and opened her own Legato Ballroom Studio in July 2020, at the height of the pandemic.

"I took a huge leap of faith," recalled Heather. "Looking back, it was the best decision I ever made. I was so grateful for the students and experiences I had before opening, which allowed me to be successful right off the bat."

As for Sarah, she wanted to continue dancing, but she no longer had male instructors. "I didn't want to be done just because I didn't have a male partner. That's wrong! I asked Heather—because I knew her and I saw what she had done with my son—if she would consider doing same-sex with me competitively. She embraced it with open arms. Yes, there were other options to find a male instructor. But here, Heather's the best. I wanted to work with the best!"

Even Luke encouraged the partnership. He told Heather, "If you can get *me* to hold my frame and posture, I'm sure you can do a lot for my mom."

Sarah and Heather developed a powerful partnership that has grown over recent years. Having a woman instructor allowed Sarah the confidence to take on the challenges of higher levels of dance and techniques.

"Men cannot replicate the way a woman's body needs to move in a rumba, swing, or cha-cha," Sarah said. "There's a whole other element that happens the longer you're in ballroom dance. You have to move in a different way than what some of our male instructors can explain. Heather can explain that physiology because she knows exactly what to say, how to move it, and where it's supposed to happen in my body. Men can make a good guess, but their bodies are not the same as ours."

For Sarah, dancing with Heather has been a great decision both as a competitive student and human being. "It's been incredible, to be honest," she said.

Sarah and Heather knew they wanted to compete as a same-sex partnership, but they also knew they needed to tell a new story through their dance. They needed it to be different from the romantic love story often created in male-female partnerships.

"We've evolved in our stylistic and choreography choices," Heather said. "At first, it was like two chicks dancing—it looked like a fad, a flash in the pan. But Sarah and I approached it from a serious competitor standpoint. We've invested in costumes that complement each other really well."

For their costumes, they created matching blue dresses. This led them to be known as "the girls in blue."

"We've invested heavily in chorography that showcases our movement as women versus choreography that is driven from a male-lead standpoint," Heather continued. "People tell us they don't like it 'when you are trying to be a dude.'"

Today, Heather's competitive students are roughly an equal mix of males and females. At some competitions, she dances professionally with females as well as with males. Sometimes the mixed performances are back-to-back.

This means she faces a special costuming challenge. She must wear a competition number on her back when leading one of her lady students, but then she must remove the number when she dances with one of her gentleman students, who all have their own numbers. It's not easy to manage those safety pins in less than thirty seconds and not hold up the competition!

The solution is literally seamless: Heather attaches her number to a specially made vest that's stoned exactly like her dress. When the same-sex dance finishes, the lady partner moves behind Heather and strips off the numbered vest just as Heather takes the arm of her gentleman partner. Done.

"Who am I to make someone wait?" Heather asked. "We want to leave same-sex competition better when we are done than when we started."

Dancing with males and females poses other unique challenges for Heather. She may have to instantly flip her routines from leader to follower. This is more complicated than it sounds because the roles are not mirror images of each other. The patterns she leads with Sarah and other ladies are "vastly different" from the patterns she follows with her gentlemen.

Why?

"Because when I'm following," Heather said, "I want to showcase my following movement. When I'm leading, I'm not trying to be a 'gentleman'—I'm trying to showcase that I can lead and still be a female."

Coaches were helpful. "Showcase your asset," they told her. "Your asset is that you *are* a woman. Show us that you know how to use your legs and hips. Own that feminine energy, and just celebrate your own power in what you're dancing."

"That makes it easy for me when I'm switching from one to the other," Heather said. "The choreography is so different."

Heather appreciates that the same-sex rule change allows women teachers to teach more lessons as well as enter in more competitions to showcase their students. Previously, women professionals could coach and train women students in their studios, but they were never allowed to competitively showcase their work.

"I had plenty of ladies who just wanted help with arm styling, hip motion, and other coaching," she said. "But they weren't consistent lessons. Why would a woman book a lesson with you when gearing for a competition, if they could never perform with you?"

Heather, forty-one, and Sarah, forty-nine, had been competing together for over four years in 2024. How have they been received on the competition dance floor?

"Sarah has had some really nice placements," Heather said. "She was a finalist at Ohio Star Ball. It's wonderful to see that judges are now marking her based on quality of dancing, versus giving her a straight last place when we started."

Straight last place?

"When we first started, leading was new to me," explained Heather. "Every good instructor should know how to lead and follow. But I never had to compete with it. There was a growth in that—in learning how to communicate well with my partner. And judges were struggling; they were like, 'It's two women out there, so we're not sure how to mark that yet.'"

Heather and the judges weren't the only ones who needed to grow when it came to same-sex dancing. A few male leaders haven't responded well out on the competition floor.

"It was almost like they said, 'I'm going to prove to you that you don't belong here,'" Heather stated. "They would make a point to dance their partner into our space. In one case, they hit us probably seven or eight times. I asked two other male professionals, 'Is it just me? Do I have to do something different with my floorcraft?' They said, 'It's not you. Dance to the side of us.' And then these two lovely gentlemen blocked the other competitor!"

Thankfully, this backlash is happening less and less as time wears on. "Generally, the top-level competitors and teachers in the country are most supportive of our same-sex dancing," Heather said.

"Once the novelty wore off, we were perceived as being serious in our dance," Sarah added.

When Heather and Sarah began competing as a same-sex couple, they were a rarity. But the number of competitive same-sex couples has grown every time they've been on the floor.

"In our Silver [intermediate] level, it was just us for a long time," Heather said. "Now we see two or three other same-sex couples. In the Bronze [initial] level, we now see five or six same-sex couples. And five or six amateur partnerships are now same-sex."

Perhaps the fact that Heather and Sarah are high-quality dance role models is a factor in that growth, both on and off the competitive dance floor. With photos of Heather and Sarah framed on the Legato Ballroom Studio walls, more amateur same-sex couples are calling their ballroom.

"Most of the partnerships are not about sexual orientation," Heather added. "There are some. But it's not the driving force."

Clearly, people are interested in same-sex dancing for many reasons. Even a mother-and-daughter team is taking lessons for an upcoming family wedding. The mother is eighty years old.

"She left me a voice message last week," Heather said with a smile. "She was saying how much they're enjoying dancing because dancing has improved her balance. She had health issues a while back. And because dance is a repetitive movement, it's not super strenuous for her. She takes the dance figures we learn and dances them in the pool to help her balance. Her daughter is just thrilled! I love seeing my seniors light up when they never thought they could do it."

I love it—mothers and daughters taking lessons together! I can't help but think about my own mother, the former Arthur Murray instructor and jitterbug queen you met in Part I, who intimidated the hell out of me for years, to the point that I was unwilling to dance. If I had only known while my mother was alive that same-sex dance could be a thing! How cool it would have been to partner with Mom for a few lessons with my young dance teacher. How lovely it would have been to share her touch and joy in something we both loved so dearly, especially as she was becoming more fragile in her aging.

Forgive me as I wipe away a tear.

Arun Garg: Quest for Quality and Tradition

At the Chicago Harvest Moon Ball in October 2023, twenty-nine-year-old Arun Garg competed in American Smooth as an advanced amateur with his professional instructor, Joseph Lettig. Joseph was the leader, Arun the follower.

As important as competing was, Arun's "number one thing" at that event was to find Alex and Kato and thank them "for everything they did." Arun didn't know them; he'd found them online when he wanted to see what a same-sex partnership might look like.

"They really hit me—this partnership works," Arun said.

He recognized that their dance movements were at the highest-quality level.

"I could not do what I do without Alex and Kato," Arun added. "Their sacrifices were instrumental. They are the ones who stripped down the barrier and tore down the wall. Without them, a lot of people would still be stuck in a mind-set that is two or three decades outdated. I have the utmost respect for them as kind and warm people who are there to uplift other artists."

Arun, who came to America from India at age three, has been breaking barriers of his own in the ballroom world, serving as role model for the newer generation. He partners not only with Joseph but also with Joseph's wife, Madalina. The husband-wife team are based in Denver, Colorado.

Arun leads Madalina in International Ballroom and follows Joseph in American Smooth. Arun dances well in both styles. But most unexpected for him was the fact that he and Joseph have made every major competition final as a same-sex couple.

"I didn't start dancing with Joseph thinking I wanted to be a champion or wanted to compete in this," Arun said. "This was supposed to be an in-house project basically to study and make me a better lead. It took off, and once the momentum was going, it was hard to say no."

His success may result in part from his lifelong immersion in music. Arun is a very serious pianist who began performing as early as middle and high school. His path to be a classical pianist was set very early in life. While taking undergraduate courses toward his chemistry and biology degrees at Mizzou, the University of Missouri, he simultaneously taught in their school of music as an adjunct faculty member and guest and contract lecturer. All at such a young age!

Arun wanted to find a social fabric and new artistic outlet in his new town of Columbia. And he found it after just one group class with the Mizzou ballroom dance club. His "dance addiction" was immediate. In just two weeks, he was breaking through a "giant newcomer field" in a collegiate dance competition, making all the final rounds. He was hooked!

In his quest to become a serious dancer, Arun began taking lessons from Larinda McRaven, a ballroom dance judge located thirty minutes south of Columbia. It was a serious introduction.

"She was so generous with her time," Arun said. "And as college kids, we were able to extract huge amounts of information that would be quite unaffordable these days."

Because the club couldn't afford professionals, Arun eventually became responsible for teaching dance basics to newer members. Larinda set very strict standards: Club members could not teach unless they really knew what they were doing. That is, they had to know both sides of the partnership—leading and following.

So Arun underwent teacher-training courses and learned to read footwork charts for both roles. That piqued his interest in dancing in a follower role.

"I can't put it specifically, but there was something psychological that felt very comforting in a follow role," he said.

After graduating college and taking a few years off for the pandemic, Arun moved to Denver, Colorado, and started dancing International Ballroom with Madalina. He knew he would be competing against young women who'd been dancing since childhood. How could he accelerate his education? Could he perhaps enlist the same successful method from Mizzou by learning the "follow rules"?

And so he started taking lessons from Joseph as a follow, creating American Smooth routines and borrowing material from his routines with Madalina. Dancing his routines with a professional man allowed him to better understand what he was asking his woman partner to do.

In June 2021, with the NDCA rule change defining a "couple" effective for just twenty months, Joseph and Arun debuted as a same-sex pro-am partnership at the Colorado Star Ball. Prepared for dead-last placements, Arun was pleasantly surprised at his results, which were confirmed by later competitions.

It is rare—and very difficult—for an amateur dancer to compete in both lead and follow roles. Why do it?

"The answer is that I love it," Arun said. "I truly love the craft of it. I'm very internally motivated. I'm a pianist, so I love the daily work. I love doing the basics, the constant drills. That fulfills my soul as an artist and keeps me happy and motivated."

I get that. But why compete as a follow in a same-sex partnership?

"First, being a follow is very enriching to one's self-image," Arun explained. "It makes you feel really good. You feel more full and more in your body because it is more external. I'm an extrovert. In many ways, I'm a performer. I'm used to being on stage alone. As a follow, you get to make every beautiful shape and be the external part of the shape. You get to fulfill pathways and be the star of it. As a leader, especially at a higher level, you start to dial back on showing that off."

To Arun, these differences between leading and following were fascinating.

"A lot has to be in relation to what your partner does," he explained. "The lead is more like preparing signals and directions and timings, so a lot of it ends up becoming smaller or more internalized. What we feel as a leader gets translated through the follow, and the follow completes it for us. So it's nice to be on the other end of it."

Arun also felt a connection to the traditional roots of ballroom dance. "After getting positive feedback from judges and colleagues for our same-sex partnership, I felt a responsibility on my shoulders and other couples' shoulders in the NDCA. I felt responsible to do it my way and do it respectfully, and to provide an example rooted in traditional quality. That's my number one thing: quality, quality, quality."

By "rooting" his movement in recognizable techniques, Arun believed his partnership would be less offensive to judges, and they could recognize that quality technical movements have nothing to do with one's sex or anything else.

"In a way," he said, "I'm a very conservative same-sex dancer because I don't switch leads in the middle of a dance. I stay the follow the whole time, and our choreography is very traditional.

We don't move away from the principles in ballroom dance that exist for a reason and that are built upon centuries of work."

Once again, Arun draws connections between his art as a dancer and as a musician. "For me, my dance is rooted in my training as a classical pianist. My entire schtick is to be conservative in that way—to conserve music that is long gone and keep it alive. I'm always looking to the past to understand layers of development that got us to where we are today. The pianism we see today is nothing like what you saw a hundred years ago. The same with ballroom dance. If you look to ballroom dance in the '90s, it is entirely different."

For Arun, respecting the traditions of the past allows him to develop a sound product that can withstand the forces of change. That's the work he feels responsible to provide—to be an example of same-sex dancing that is palatable to even the most resistant opinions within the NDCA.

"When that lawsuit happened, it didn't necessarily change minds," Arun said, referring to Carol Lockwood's rule-changing lawsuit, described earlier in this chapter. "People were still going to have their opinions. It takes time to change. And it takes actual, tangible change to really enforce that across the culture. That's the work I feel responsible to do. I feel responsible to provide a consistent quality in a traditionally recognizable partnership so judges aren't looking at gender but can focus on really good movement. That's what I want to portray. For me, it's not really a gender story at all."

And though Arun is a gay man, he says that's not his focus when it comes to same-sex dancing. "My focus is so far apart from the gender or sensual side of it. I'm focused on the mechanics and how to build myself as a dancer."

How has Arun and Joseph's same-sex partnership been received?

"Right off the bat," Arun said, "some judges were worried about how the clientele would take it. How would the pro-am ladies feel about dancing against a man? But I found from day one, without exception, that there has been nothing but love and acceptance, celebration and support from my colleagues in the pro-am division. They don't treat me any different. They treat me very well. I've never felt outcast by any of my co-competitors, by any other lady or guy. I feel like family. It's been really positive."

Well, it wasn't *all* rosy, he admitted. At least one male professional dancing pro-am with a female student has intentionally interfered with Arun and Joseph on the competition dance floor, similar to Heather and Sarah's experience.

"To me, that's just a sign that the other person is insecure," Arun observed.

As for the future, Arun continues to teach and lecture around the country as a classical pianist and musician. He has become more involved in the ballroom dance competition industry itself, often working for competition organizers in various senior administrative roles, such as registrar or scrutineer. That allows him to compete pro-am "as long as I live."

Currently, he works at a competition almost every other weekend. The dance-based travel provides him opportunities to also give lectures and take on teaching engagements around the country. He has no interest in turning professional himself or in competing in a professional partnership.

Arun is most happy to see other same-sex partnerships "giving their own spin on it and flooding the market. If it's just one person, you can't make institutional change," he said. "You can't force eyes to see anything different. It has to be a barrage of people, a mass of people who are committed long-term with quality behind their dancing. That's the biggest thing."

For Arun, the experience has been incredibly empowering. "I'm both pleasantly surprised and actually shocked at how well it's gone, compared to what people warned me it would be like three years ago, when I first started. I'm in a place in my ballroom dancing and in the ballroom industry I never would have thought. I have personal relationships with heroes of mine I never thought I would have access to, even as a student. So it really has been a very positive experience."

A Personal Note: From Breakdown to Breakthrough

I'm grateful to all the people who chose to share their personal stories of resilience for this book, but I extend a special word of thanks to the storytellers who shared for this chapter. I learned much from them about the kind of resilience it takes to change an entire industry steeped in tradition.

Don't get me wrong—same-sex dancing has long existed. Other dance groups have welcomed same-sex partners in both social and competitive venues over the years. Take country dancers, for example. Or nightclub dancers, such as fans of West Coast Swing. They've led the way.

But for some reason, those groups' informality regarding partnerships never broke through to the conservative realm of traditional ballroom dance. People like the storytellers in this chapter had to battle for change in the world of ballroom dance.

As Arun shared, one person can't make institutional change. As one person, you can't force eyes to see anything different. You can change rules. But only a "mass" of people can change minds.

And yes, minds *are* changing in the ballroom world today. We can celebrate that.

Frankly, the ballroom world has lagged behind the political world. I remember the controversy and pushback I received in 1993 when, as a Minnesota state senator, I voted for state human rights policies prohibiting discrimination against gays and lesbians. The legislation passed. Two weeks later, I was picketed at a town hall meeting in my suburban Minneapolis senate district. It was the only time that happened in my eighteen-year senate career.

In the end, it wasn't our legislative change that caused institutional change. Change happened at the institutional level only after it happened in the hearts and minds of our constituents. As more people identified themselves as gays and lesbians, we discovered they were our neighbors, our colleagues, and, yes, our own family members. We already knew them as human beings. Nothing really changed in our relationships.

In 2012, long after I retired from the senate, Minnesota conservatives proposed a ballot initiative that would make clear that marriage in our state was between a man and a woman. That hard-fought political battle around the anti-marriage amendment mobilized what was then known as the LGBT community and their allies in ways never seen before. Minnesota voters were the first in the country to reject such an initiative.

And the unexpected result was yet to come. Just one year later, public opinion regarding LGBT rights was such that the legislature could pass a law *making same-sex marriage legal.* What a turnaround in hearts and minds in just one year!

The NDCA rule change occurred nearly a decade after legislatures like ours wrestled with these issues. Even then, it took a two-year-long legal "breakdown" to cause fundamental change. But from breakdown comes breakthrough. The storytellers in this chapter helped create it.

No, not all hearts and minds in the traditional ballroom dance world have accepted same-sex partnerships yet. But momentum grows every year. I expect we'll see significant competitive involvement of same-sex partnerships in the future.

Just as we observed in Minnesota politics, change is happening in the dance world as same-sex partners come forward and as we get to know these men and women. They are our friends. They are our fellow professionals and students. And we all share one thing in common—a deep love for the art of quality dance.

Dance on!

Chapter 24

⌄

Suni Lee: Shining Gold on the Hmong Community

We turn now to the story of two remarkable women from different generations who broke through years of history to shine a light on a cultural community that no longer had a place to call home. These women are members of the Lee clan of the Hmong community in Saint Paul, Minnesota. And yes, they're both ballroom dancers.

Choua Lee, now in her mid-fifties, was the first Hmong person ever elected to public office in the United States. She accomplished that at the tender age of twenty-three. She served on the Saint Paul school board for six years.

And Suni Lee, at just eighteen years old, made *Hmong* the single-most-searched word on global social media the day she won the 2021 Olympic gold medal for all-around gymnastics in Tokyo. The world wanted to know more.

Both women shone a light on a nearly forgotten Southeast Asian culture. That light is still shining. After Suni's Tokyo success, Choua and her husband, Cheu, commissioned a mural in Suni's honor on a building they own in Saint Paul. They also helped produce a video for the song "Suni Lee" by artist Lil Crush.

And Suni Lee went on to again surprise the world when she recovered from debilitating kidney disease and rallied at the Paris 2024 Olympics, where she won team gold and two individual bronze medals. Not to mention that Suni excelled as a celebrity dancer on *Dancing with the Stars* in fall 2021, immediately after the Tokyo games. Resilience!

Hmong women and families are shaped by their dramatic history. Choua still has "vivid memories" of leaving Laos in 1976 at age seven, along with her parents and older sister. As American allies, they had to leave Southeast Asia after the Fall of Saigon and the end of the Vietnam War. Her family traveled on foot for weeks to get out of the country. They slept outdoors without shelter, even during pouring rain.

"We learned to adapt," Choua said. "We learned to survive. That's what shaped my generation. Any aspiration comes from the need to survive, to work hard, and excel. You must do whatever it takes to adapt to your environment. There are no other options. You *have* to do it."

But along the way, there is always hope.

"That's the resiliency," Choua continued. "My mom never wasted time trying to calm us down. She told us we would do well, that we would go to America, where we would have enough food and water and basic necessities. How did she know? She just knew. She was a woman beyond her time."

Choua was raised in Chicago and Saint Paul, and she eventually attended what was then known as Mankato State University in Minnesota. There she met Cheu and married him in 1989. She left college as a junior to work as the director of a Hmong women's organization for two years.

Through that advocacy work, Choua witnessed firsthand the struggles Hmong and other immigrant parents were having with the school district. She brought that to the attention of a Minnesota state senator, who urged her to run citywide for the Saint Paul school board.

Two weeks after Choua jumped into the school board race, she learned she was pregnant. That didn't stop her. The

195

twenty-three-year-old gave birth seven days after being sworn into office in 1991. Minnesota and the nation took notice of this new Hmong official, who had just been elected by the people of Saint Paul.

Talk about adaptability, survival, and resiliency!

Those same qualities drove Choua into ballroom dance many years later. Dance had been her passion since the age of two. She found clever ways to learn classical Thai dance in Laos. When she was only four years old, she stood outside an open-air classroom and observed the dance lessons.

Later, at age ten in Chicago, she bartered English lessons for classical Thai dance lessons with a nursing student who was also a Thai dancer. Thai dance was all Choua knew because Hmong culture does not recognize ballroom dance. In traditional Laos dance, partners dance side by side with no contact; there is no lead-and-follow.

That all changed when Choua joined a youth dance group arising from a nonprofit her parents had created to support refugee resettlement. Her group performed at a community center, where she saw ballroom dancers for the first time.

"The moment I saw the ballroom costumes, the rhinestones, and the flowing of the gowns, my world turned upside down," she recalled. "I knew deep inside that I was going to do that one day. I promised myself, but I didn't know how. I fell in love with ballroom."

As the years progressed, Choua and Cheu busied themselves with work and family. They knew little else. There was no time for hobbies such as dance. But then life changed when their son left to attend boarding school in Thailand.

"I remember we were both alone at home," Choua recalled. "We were in different rooms watching different programs. We had to do something!"

Choua finally saw an opportunity to revisit her dream of ballroom dance. It was no dream for Cheu, though. He couldn't dance, he said. He thought ballroom was for girls.

But for Choua, there was "no other option." She reserved

two free sessions with instructor Dustin Donelan at Cinema Ballroom and repeated over and over to Cheu, "We are dancing Thursday." She wore him out.

"Cheu was so nervous he couldn't breathe," Choua recalled of their first lessons. "My assertive side kept coming out to 'rescue' both of us. I wanted to lead and take charge, like everything else. Dustin was so good. He told me, 'You can't do that. Close your eyes. Feel it. Don't take control.' Finally, Dustin threatened to blindfold me. Cheu couldn't lead because I was so controlling. I wouldn't let him grow. So for a few weeks, I danced with my eyes closed. Then I let go. Cheu's skills just grew. He started loving it."

The couple dived in. They took a lesson or group class nearly every day: class at seven o'clock, home by eight thirty, practice until midnight. They cleared kitchen space and practiced at least two hours every night.

"After two years, I decided this was something for which the Hmong community needed exposure," Choua continued. "So I made it my mission. I researched how ballroom came to be, and I brought in other Hmong. I learned how to lead and follow. We were able to generate interest in the community of empty nesters. At one point, we had about twenty couples coming weekly. The group created the Hmong American Ballroom Society in 2010, which influenced Hmong dance groups in other states."

So, did Choua's love of ballroom dancing influence Suni Lee to compete on *Dancing with the Stars*? No. Though Choua and Cheu are designated as grandparents of Suni within the Lee clan, they do not have a biological relationship with her. They have, of course, supported her gymnastic efforts over the years as funders and as cheerleaders.

"*Dancing with the Stars* was really her decision," Choua said. "Fellow gymnast Simone Biles, a past dancer on the show, was a big influence. They spent a lot of time together. Suni didn't have a social life. She'd been in grueling training since age five or six. She's always in the gym, always traveling. She just wanted to take some time off and not compete in gymnastics for a time. I was surprised when she decided to compete on *Dancing with the Stars*. She insisted on having some fun."

So how did Suni do during her dancing debut, in the eyes of her ballroom-trained grandparents?

"I think she did a great job, since she didn't have formal training in ballroom," Choua said with a smile. "She had stamina, flexibility, and gymnastics prowess. The first few weeks, she struggled with the rhythm of the dance, not the gymnastics side. She was new to the format and pace of the dance. She tended to catch up on timing and forget the rhythm. But she showed great improvement as the weeks progressed."

Another hurdle for Suni was the demonstrative nature of ballroom dance. That type of self-expression was hard for Choua, too, when she competed in ballroom competitions.

"Hmong society tends to be more introverted," Choua explained. "We don't like to be too loud or too extroverted. That is frowned upon. Girls don't want to be too flamboyant. Hmong girls are demure and proper. Body language is proper. Gymnastics fit right into that, but dance is different. It's hard for us to show external expression. I remember the first year I competed in ballroom—my instructor told me I needed more expression. He told me to 'triple-time' my expression for the audience to see it. I think Suni has a hard time with that too."

Suni placed in the semifinals of her *Dancing with the Stars* competition. But her Olympic-sized impact continued to ripple through world cultures on multiple levels.

"Suni reached a pivotal point in excellency," Choua said. "I think her achievements are going to change the younger generation for years to come. I already hear things in the Hmong community like, 'I'm so happy. She looks like me. I can do it now.' Isn't that great? I also hear from non-Hmong girls, 'I'm so happy! I want to be like Suni Lee!' It's just amazing to hear something like this. I don't think we'll realize the impact of her winning or the impact of her achievement on the community until the next fifty years. I don't think Suni herself fully understands the impact or significance of her wins."

Fifty years? Really?

"I didn't think I would see this in my lifetime," Choua continued. "From the time of the war and struggle in Laos, we experienced trauma. What's all of that for? For the betterment of our society, of being recognized, of being on the world stage. It took thousands of lives, soldiers, family sacrifices, the ultimate sacrifice, and we haven't even achieved that level. And here's this little girl who went to Tokyo, and she has overcome that. The world wants to know who the Hmong people are. That is such an achievement. You talk about General Vang Pao—the sacrifices he and others made for fifty or sixty years. They haven't even come close to what Suni did. Suni elevated the Hmong people to the world stage. That's something we should all celebrate. It's amazing. It's that power, that power alone."

According to Choua, it's not only a cultural breakthrough but a gender breakthrough as well.

"A little girl rose to that level, even when women are being so oppressed in society. You talk with any Hmong woman, and she can tell you stories about personal suffering through years of abuse, oppression, you name it. Now Hmong women are telling their stories. They had to be the strong one, raise a family, be a role model for their children, and make sure their children had shelter and food on the table every single day."

Talk about resilience. Two extraordinary women driven by excellence and hard work, adapting to whatever stands in their way. Adaptation is their inspiration. It's rooted in a need to survive. And it's rooted in hope.

These are the values that served Choua and Suni well. They're values that serve all of us well—whether we're navigating the ballroom dance floor or navigating the crucibles life sends our way.

Chapter 25

❧

Dancers Lead in Creating
New Cultural Norms

D r. Don DeBoer chose not to create his own practice as a licensed psychologist but instead has engaged students in talk therapy for over fifteen years at Saint Paul's Macalester College. When he leaves the campus health clinic at night, he teaches salsa and Latin dance at a local studio. That feeds his soul and his multiethnic roots.

"I feel like teaching dance is my private practice," he said. "I like it better. The dance I'm doing is therapy—no doubt about that—though it's not necessarily 'dance therapy.' I'm not formally trained as a dance/movement therapist or an expressive arts therapist. But to me, it doesn't matter, as long as you're getting therapeutic value out of it. There is this undeniable connection between psychotherapy and the arts. My training as a dancer and as a psychologist were always two different things, but they always happened concurrently for me."

Don can relate to the trials of the college students he counsels. In high school, he wasn't confident, and he didn't feel "smart enough." He wasn't an achiever.

"I was probably depressed off and on and a little lonely," he recalled.

Today, he might say he suffered from imposter syndrome, where one's confidence level doesn't match their accomplishments or station. But his mother encouraged him to go to college, and now Don encourages students with his own experience.

"It's not about whether you're talented or not," he said. "Or whether you're smart or not. For me, it boiled down to this: Do you want to put the work into it? And if you're absolutely passionate about it, then you'll get to where you're going, and you'll finally be there."

He feels the same way about dance. "With the right attitude and encouragement and patience, people will get there. And quite frankly, when you love art, you just have to do it. I like people to realize these things are more attainable than they realize."

Don's interest in dance came from his love of music and his multiethnicity. Music is his lifeline. It has always connected him to people and made him happy.

After high school, he thought he could be a DJ, so he enrolled at a community college and took classes in radio and television communications. He also took speech courses to overcome his shyness. As he excelled in communications, he gained confidence and began to overcome his imposter syndrome. In time, he realized he'd always wanted to be a psychologist, though he'd never considered himself smart enough. He transferred to a four-year university to pursue psychology.

Meanwhile, he volunteered as a DJ at a local radio station and loved hearing the Latin rhythms. It bothered him that he was part Puerto Rican and didn't know how to dance to Latin music. Dance was tied to his cultural identity, which made it more important to him to invest in it.

Though Don's father is of Dutch descent, his mother is of Puerto Rican and Indigenous Hawaiian descent. Don was born in Hawaii, and while he was raised and attended college in Washington state, he spent his summers in Hawaii with his mother's side of the family. His grandmother grew up in an era when one was embarrassed to be Hawaiian. At that time one could not even speak Hawaiian lest they be considered "less than." She became an activist who started the Office of Hawaiian Affairs.

"That's why those cultural elements are important to me and why I didn't want to assimilate completely," Don said. "I think when you come from a people that's been marginalized and colonized, whatever you have left, you know how precious it is. You preserve it. So my grandmother was always instilling that in me and telling me that my Puerto Rican and Hawaiian side was special. She told me I should be proud."

When Don moved to the Twin Cities in 1993 to pursue his PhD in counseling psychology at the University of Minnesota, he missed his Puerto Rican and Hawaiian family members, so he immediately sought out the Latino community. It gave him a sense of identity, comfort, and family.

"When you're an American citizen and you're multiethnic, you have a more complex understanding of cultural identity," he said. "There's the irony that you're exploring a culture that you're already supposed to be in. There's a dissonance between fitting in and not fitting in. At the same time, people assume you want to blend in completely to the white culture, so why bother to make a fuss over the other parts of your cultural identity?"

Music and ethnicity led Don to his eventual "home" in the Twin Cities' Latino dance community. Depressed at the breakup of a relationship, Don decided to take a salsa dance class with a friend in a similar situation.

"I think we quit after the first day," he recalled. "I couldn't keep up. It seemed like everybody was ahead of me."

(Kind of like those old high school days?)

Overwhelmed by the class, Don got a "how to dance salsa" VHS tape. So, he had the tape, he had Latin music from his radio days, he had a partner, and he had a passion for breaking things down. The pair learned on their own, went back to the class, and were better than everyone else.

"Again, it's my philosophy," Don said. "It's just the work. Study it. A lot of people thought that was funny. Counting, counting! Taking notes. How else am I supposed to learn this stuff?"

Don never knew the ballroom crowd. Everything he did was through the Latin dance nightclub culture. For Don, dance has never been a competitive thing. What he loves most about dancing in the Latin culture is the sense of bonding and inclusion.

"It belongs to everybody," he said. "It's supposed to be a community thing."

Around 1995–96, Don started lessons with Rebecca Abas of Four Seasons Dance Studio in Minneapolis.

"She was the only one at the time teaching salsa the way that Latinos were actually doing it," he said. "I became addicted."

At one point, he danced about twelve hours per week between lessons, group classes, video practice, and nightclubs.

"I became a fanatic, and I lost about thirty pounds," he said. "For the first time, I was aware of my body in ways I wasn't aware before. I was cultivating my look. I was meeting people. It was a natural antidepressant. I was connecting to culture, connecting to music, connecting to people. What a high that was! And coming from a psychologist's standpoint, this to me was like medicine. Why have people talk to me about their problems and get prescribed antidepressants when they could be going out and exercising, enjoying culture, and meeting people? To me, this was a gift waiting for me. It just felt right. There were things I could do with my body that no one ever taught me. It just came out. I would wonder, 'Is that in my DNA?'"

In 1998 Rebecca invited him to teach at Four Seasons. He has since taught salsa classes weekly there for over twenty-five years, including teaching by Zoom during the pandemic.

"I like analyzing dance because I want to know what the rules are," he explained. "For me, that's the joy of teaching because I'm looking at movement and I'm deriving rules and order out of this beautiful visual phenomenon. We add numbers to that. And this pause. This beat's longer than that. I love that part of it. That might be different than somebody who likes movement in an abstract, freeform way."

Along the way, Don also taught classes in various nightclubs, including a gay nightclub in downtown Minneapolis called the Saloon.

"We were going to do a Latin night," Don said, "and I was excited because the gay Latinos couldn't go anywhere to dance without people gawking at us. I was warned by the club manager that it might not fly. Well, they underestimated. The first night we had salsa at the Saloon, tons of gay and lesbian Latinos were there."

From that point on, Don taught an LGBT salsa class for years.

"In the past, you had to have a 'gay night.' That changed. The fact that you didn't need a 'night' anymore says a lot about our progress. A gay couple could go to any nightclub and dance together and wouldn't be treated terribly or gawked at. Hopefully, gays and lesbians have become mainstream enough that you don't need a separate dance night to have fun."

Perhaps. In 2023, Don was again hired to teach an LGBT salsa class. Attendance boomed after the second election of President Donald Trump. "Progress and backlash apparently continue to exist side by side," he said.

Don's main focus, however, continues to be his two careers: psychotherapy and dance. They are therapeutic in different ways.

"I love talk therapy because I do consider myself verbal and intellectual," he said. "And the students are that way as well. They are learners. But dance was therapeutic in a way I didn't appreciate with talk therapy. When you're in talk therapy, you're talking about things. When you're dancing, you're just *in* it. There's something subversive about it. It's very present. It feels like a rush of positive energy throughout your body. Pretty powerful. Almost like an addiction, but a positive addiction. It feels more wholistic, maybe. When I'm in talk therapy, I'm this talking head. But when I'm dancing, my whole body is in there. And there's touch involved—that's also powerful."

Don stayed grounded during the pandemic by imagining the future "rebirth" of the dance scene. As the pandemic resolved and social activity slowly resumed, people risked taking private lessons.

"They told me it helped," Don said. "You could see in their faces—they were just elated. So thankful. It's like the pandemic said, 'I'm taking away all of your toys, and I'm not giving them back until you really appreciate them.' Start thinking about gratitude. Start thinking about hope."

Gratitude and hope may well secure the foundation for the dance community for years to come. Wouldn't that be the best therapy of all . . . for us all?

Chapter 26

‿

A Powerful Presence in
the Ballroom World

On May 25, 2020, George Floyd was murdered in Minneapolis, just a few miles away from me. Civil unrest followed in our city and around the country, turning a spotlight on racial injustice and discrimination.

In the wake of Floyd's death, I reached out to my longtime friend and former dance teacher, Nathan Daniels, also of Minneapolis. I wanted to talk about things we rarely talked about.

I knew a lot about Nathan, of course. I knew that he was one of only four African American men who were certified ballroom dance judges in North America. (This is out of about seven hundred total judges and fifty-four judges of color.)

I knew that Nathan could have been anything he wanted to be before he chose a life of dance. I knew that he'd graduated from Duke University (our shared alma mater) at twenty years old with a BA in sociology and economics and minors in premed and prelaw. I knew that he'd made a greater impact as a dance professional and role model than he ever could have made in another profession.

Most importantly, I knew that he was direct, self-confident, and quick to cut through excuses. I also knew that he was fun, witty, and well liked in the ballroom world.

But there was much I didn't know about him—much I wanted to learn now. So I asked him, how does an African American man born in the South survive in a ballroom dance world that has been essentially white for decades? Has he—or does he—experience discrimination as a dance professional? And what has been his experience with racism as a black man in a lifelong partnership with Michael, a white man?

Nathan's responses surprised me. His experiences and internal struggles were almost opposite of what I'd envisioned. Of course, my expectations were bound by my white experience; I'd assumed that he'd faced many more overt obstacles relating to his race.

Nathan's story began in Virginia and North Carolina, where he lived during his early years. His father always worked in occupations that helped children, earning a master's degree in social and vocational rehabilitation counseling. Nathan's mother was a teacher with a master's in home economics. Their fifty-three-year marriage was a great foundation for Nathan. So was their commitment to education.

"I have a brain," Nathan told me. "There was never a question that I would be educated or go to a fine school. That's how it was. Education can never be taken away from you."

Nathan's parents provided him with key life education as well.

"My parents prepared me for living in a white world, without actually saying it," he said. "They taught me that the manner of talk and dress and even the kind of car you drive were all instrumental to how you behave. 'This is what you need to do to not be considered a thug,' they told me. My father was an eloquent speaker. He always corrected my words."

Nathan's parents gave him such great self-esteem that he couldn't fathom that someone wouldn't like him or discriminate against him.

"My parents told me, 'You're great! You can do whatever you want. You have a great brain!' Those were the rose-colored glasses I had on. In general, I haven't had a lot of overt racism in my life. I saw racism in the South, but I didn't know that's what it was. I would hear 'white people' or 'colored people.' I was not consciously affected by it because my little brain wouldn't go there."

But racism did affect the family, even if young Nathan was not conscious of it. His mom was light-skinned and could pass for white, so Nathan's parents were accused of having an interracial relationship, causing jeers and discomfort.

When Nathan was about eight years old, the family moved to New York to start a better life for him. Nathan doubts life was "better" there; it was maybe just "surface nice." But again, he was too young to grasp such things.

Nathan graduated from Duke in the spring of 1978 and planned to attend Stanford Law School in the fall. That summer, he returned to New York City and spent hours and hours dancing in nightclubs. The Hustle was the rage at the time.

One night, a guy approached him. "You're really good," he said to Nathan. "Have you ever thought about going into the dance business? I have a studio. Why not come down and see what it's about?"

Six intense weeks later, with eight hours a day split between dance training and sales training, Nathan was a dance teacher. So much for law school. He immediately launched his professional dance career, and he never looked back.

"I just fell in love with it," Nathan recalled. "It was a calling for me—this makes me happy. It was a healthy lifestyle, plus you were helping other people, giving them something they needed. The level of your dancing didn't matter to people. As long as you were charismatic, they liked you, and you made them happy."

Nathan earned $3.50 an hour plus 2 percent commission on any dance lessons he sold. He taught the Hustle forty hours a week, more than anyone else in his training class. Still, it was far from lucrative. The only way he could manage was to live at home. He received free dance training from the studio so he could stay one step ahead of his students.

Thankfully, Nathan was cloaked in self-confidence, so he never had trouble gaining or keeping students. He earned respect as a high-caliber teacher when six of his women students earned championships in national competitions.

Nathan moved to Minneapolis in 1990. He and his professional dance partner, Deanne Michael, began competing in the theater arts category, which includes complex lifts. They went on to win the United States Rising Star Theatre Arts Championship.

Over the years, Nathan built a reputation as both a good teacher and good dancer. The idea of becoming a judge never crossed his mind until 2002, when he realized he didn't want to compete professionally anymore.

Deciding out of the blue to become a judge was a bit of a disadvantage. As Nathan explained, there's a "pecking order" in how judges get hired for competitions and events, in part based on their specific dance career experience. Had he known earlier that he wanted to become a judge, he would have made different decisions as a dancer.

Despite taking a unique route to judging, Nathan finally got a taste of the experience when he was invited to perform in Canada and judge as well. He went on to pass his exams and qualify as a US championship judge in all five dance divisions.

Now in his mid-sixties, Nathan has judged over two hundred dance competitions throughout the United States. National rankings show that his judging scores track highly with final placements in competitions. He is known for his impartiality and his focus on technique, especially technique in footwork.

When you are one of only four African American male judges in the country, your mere presence makes an impact. A few years ago, Nathan judged a competition in Baton Rouge, Louisiana. The local school superintendent attended the event to support his students, and he made a point to approach Nathan.

"You have no idea what your presence means here," the superintendent said. "The kids are just in awe that someone could rise to that level because they haven't seen it before."

Nathan also gets attention when he volunteers his time to judge school competitions in the Dancing Classrooms program (see Chapter 16). "I can do that!" ten-year-old Harry, also African American, told him. These young students see Nathan's confidence—the confidence his parents instilled in him. And now Nathan can pass that confidence on to the younger generation.

But while Nathan's confident presence and quality judging made an impact on the dance floor, the world changed around him. For years, his "rose-colored glasses" had seemingly shielded him from overt racism in his career and his community. But the glasses were slowly coming off.

When Nathan was a teen, his parents had given him "The Talk" that black boys often receive to prepare for interactions with police. Despite this, he still held a very positive image of the police for years. He had friends and family in law enforcement, and he'd only ever been stopped by Minnesota police for normal traffic violations. It hadn't entered his mind that police could be bad.

That is, until he served on a Minneapolis jury for a murder case in the mid-1990s. The defendant was clearly guilty, but the jury had to acquit him because the police had done "a really bad job." The case redirected his thinking.

Though Nathan was told there was racism in Minneapolis, he hadn't experienced it firsthand. So around 1996, he decided to test it with his life partner, Michael, a white man. They chose to shop in a prominent men's clothing store, with Nathan shopping first on his own and Michael shopping on his own about five minutes later.

"We had two totally different experiences," Nathan recalled. "I was followed around the store the entire time. It wasn't in a 'May I help you?' way. They definitely wanted to keep an eye on me. Michael wasn't followed at all. We were dressed the same, walked the same route in the store, and observed the same three people at the register."

What does Nathan think today, after multiple incidents of black people being treated differently and sometimes tragically, like in the cases of Breonna Taylor and George Floyd? Nathan admits that he now lives a more realistic, "rose-colored-glasses-off" existence. Every time he goes out his door, he knows he must be careful. He doesn't walk in certain neighborhoods at certain times. He doesn't leave without his phone or ID. He doesn't wear baggy jeans or a hoodie.

"It's sad to lose that naïveté," he said. "That's the world we live in. I don't have any qualms about saying that now because that is my reality."

And this brings Nathan to an ethical dilemma in his current ballroom dance career. For years, he received multiple invitations for judging panels around the country, due to his work product and reputation. But things change and the offers are fewer now. The new generation of dancers doesn't know him, especially the many dancers and judges who come from other countries. It's difficult for Nathan to gain more exposure because he's an independent professional with no studio affiliation, he doesn't organize a competition, and he's not a recent former champion.

Nathan's request to obtain the highest certification as a national judge has been denied—twice—because he doesn't meet all the qualifications. Yet several other people who don't meet the qualifications have been certified as national judges due to "specific circumstances."

Is Nathan experiencing racial discrimination in the ballroom world, after all these years? "Being the person I am, I err on the side of positivity, that it is not racially motivated at all," he said. "My brain won't let me go there. I'd be very disheartened if that was the case."

Despite these recent challenges, Nathan knows that his presence as a black professional judge on the dance floor is still important. He would love to compose a résumé that says, "You need to hire me because you need more people of color on your panel. You want to increase the dance business, and there's an entire untapped market, but you're not going to get it unless they see people like them in positions of authority."

He knows that his presence gives hope and confidence to others, particularly in these sensitive times. He knows that he is a good judge. So, he asks himself, should he market himself in a way to increase diversity within the judging panel? Should he use his platform of ethnicity to attain national certification under a "specific circumstance"? Or will it appear that he is requesting special treatment because he is black?

"I'm in a precarious situation here," he admitted. "I'm basically saying, 'Hire me because I'm black, not because I'm qualified.' But I *am* qualified. So I don't know whether that's the avenue I want to go down. It's a conundrum. What if they say no? I'll never know if being black is the reason or not. I don't know whether I want blackness to be one of those 'special circumstances.' Once I do this, there's no going back because it'll be nationally known that's what I did."

I said earlier that Nathan's story surprised me. This part of his story perhaps surprised me most of all. In my own experience as a white woman, I have eagerly and intentionally advocated for more leadership opportunities for myself and other women and girls. Yet here is Nathan, unsure whether to use his blackness as an advancement opportunity for himself and, more importantly, for others.

But I get it—times are changing. Identity politics are less in the forefront. We saw that in how Vice President Kamala Harris approached the 2024 presidential campaign. And regretfully, we have seen it even more in the second administration of President Donald J. Trump, where the rollback of diversity, equity, and inclusion is a top priority, and where corporations and other organizations around the country feel pressure to follow suit, even as marginalized identities face greater challenges.

But black lives *do* matter in community and in the ballroom dance world. Nathan's life of strength and accomplishment is a beacon of hope not only for black individuals but for everyone else as well. He is a role model for future generations, and he just happens to be black.

We need that now, more than ever.

PART V

Dance Science: Medicine for the Aging Body, Mind, and Soul

Frequent dance is 76 percent more effective than any other form of exercise in preventing dementia. Dance lowers the risk of depression and the risk of some cancers and cardiovascular diseases. Dance can reduce and may slow down the progression of Parkinson's disease (PD) symptoms and improve problem-solving abilities.

In the following pages, specialized dance professionals, dance medicine practitioners, and a dance movement therapist personally share their experiences with the interplay between medical science, brain health, and dance benefits for all ages. They know firsthand how dance becomes even more impactful to our physical, emotional, and mental health as we age.

Chapter 27

◆

The Science Behind the
Healthier, Happier Dancer

Throughout this book, you've met storytellers who experienced—and now practically evangelize—the health benefits of dance. Dance created better posture for some dancers. It was an antidote to depression for grieving spouses. It improved endurance and body tone for large and small dancers alike. Then there was the surgeon who danced his way out of needing a knee replacement. And there was Jim, who used dance to reconnect his leg to his brain after being gored by a buffalo.

These are all amazing examples of the power of dance. But the benefits of dance go well beyond this.

"Promoting Physical Activity to Patients," a September 2019 study in the *British Medical Journal*, found that regular dancing lowered the risk of dementia and depression by 20 to 30 percent. There were other physical benefits as well: It lowered the risk of colon cancer by 30 percent, lowered the risk of breast cancer by 20 percent, and lowered the risk of cardiovascular disease by 20 to 30 percent.[1]

In 2023, US Surgeon General Dr. Vivek H. Murthy issued *Our Epidemic of Loneliness and Isolation: The U.S. Surgeon*

General's Advisory on the Healing Effects of Social Connection and Community. It concluded that loneliness and social isolation represent profound threats to our health and well-being.

The advisory cited key data showing that loneliness and social isolation increase the risk for premature death by 26 percent and 29 percent, respectively. But what attracted the biggest headlines was the surgeon general's announcement that "lack of social connection can increase the risk for premature death as much as smoking up to 15 cigarettes a day."

That wasn't all. The cited data also showed that poor or insufficient social connection is associated with increased risk for anxiety, depression, and dementia and may increase susceptibility to viruses and respiratory illness. The latter might seem counterintuitive to most of us, as we normally associate social connections with health risks due to contagion.

Finally, the advisory data showed that lack of social connection was associated with a 29 percent increased risk of heart disease and a 32 percent increased risk of stroke. Wow.

Of course, all these health risks come with economic costs to individuals and community. The surgeon general cited data that social isolation among older adults alone accounts for an estimated $6.7 billion in excess Medicare spending annually, largely due to increased hospital and nursing facility spending.

So, just how prevalent are social isolation and loneliness? More than you may think. The advisory cited surveys showing that approximately half of adults in the United States report experiencing loneliness, with some of the highest rates among young adults. Loneliness is generally defined as the subjective internal state of distress when an individual's actual experience differs from a preferred experience.

Even more concerning was a 2022 study, cited in the advisory, that found that only 39 percent of adults in the United States indicated that they felt socially connected to others. That means many adults feel socially isolated, objectively defined as having few social relationships or group activities and infrequent social interaction.

According to the advisory, social isolation and loneliness are more widespread than many other major health issues of the day, including smoking (12.5 percent of adults), diabetes (14.7 percent), and obesity (41.0 percent), with comparable levels of risk to health and premature death. Yet less than 20 percent of individuals who often or always feel lonely recognize it as a major problem.[2]

Now that's a public health crisis.

Engaging in movement and partner dance is at least a partial antidote to many of the health issues described above. But of all the benefits of partner dance highlighted in the literature, one stands out as the most profound: It can bring new life to seniors confronting difficult neurological challenges such as dementia and Parkinson's disease.

Take the 2003 landmark study of senior citizens over age seventy-five, led by the Albert Einstein College of Medicine in New York City and reported in the *New England Journal of Medicine*. The study demonstrated that frequent dancing provides the greatest risk reduction of dementia of any activity studied, cognitive or physical.

The study was described by Richard Powers in "Use It or Lose It: Dancing Makes You Smarter, Longer." The researchers evaluated the subjects' cognitive activities such as reading books, writing for pleasure, doing crossword puzzles, playing cards, and playing musical instruments over a twenty-one-year period. They also studied the subjects' physical activities such as playing tennis or golf, swimming, bicycling, dancing, walking for exercise, and doing housework.

Check out these results: Reading lowered dementia risk by 35 percent, and working crossword puzzles at least four days per week reduced dementia risk by 47 percent. Tennis, golf, swimming, bicycling, walking, and housework didn't appear to offer any protection against dementia.

As for frequent partner dancing? Of *all* the activities studied, it yielded the greatest reduction of dementia risk, by 76 percent.

Let's say that again: *by 76 percent!*

According to the study, this protective benefit stems from the complexity of dance and the effect it has on neural pathways. As people age, random brain cells die. And if someone has only one well-worn pathway in the brain, it can be completely blocked when certain cells die. "But those who spent their lives trying different mental routes each time, creating a myriad of possible paths, still have several paths left," Powers wrote. Dance helps create such pathways.

Do all forms of dancing provide the same protective benefits? No. Dance that merely focuses on style or retraces the same memorized paths does not. While Powers conceded that dance, in general, can reduce stress and provide cardiovascular and socialization benefits, he stressed that "the more decision-making we can bring into our dancing, the better." And those benefits are greatly enhanced when we dance with different partners.[3, 4]

What does "decision-making" mean? Whether you are a leader or follower, partner dance involves split-second, rapid-fire decision-making. In partner dance, you each make choices. Even when choreographed, partner dance doesn't rely on rote memory or focus only on physical style. It's not automatic. It requires active intelligence and attention.

The importance of this finding cannot be underestimated. A study published in *Nature Medicine* on January 13, 2025, found the lifetime risk of dementia after age fifty-five to be 42 percent. Rates were substantially higher in women and black adults. The number of US adults who will develop dementia each year was projected to double, from about 514,000 in 2020 to approximately 1 million adults in 2060.[5]

Dementia isn't the only neurological condition for which dance creates a profound impact. As early as 2007, a group of physiotherapists found that when people with Parkinson's disease danced in a series of partnered tango classes, they experienced great improvement in their physical symptoms. Dance psychologist Dr. Peter Lovatt tested these results for himself through a study of people living with Parkinson's who participated in ten sessions of contact improvisation dance. He observed not only physical improvement but emotional and cognitive improvement as well.[6]

David Leventhal, a cofounder of the Mark Morris Dance Group's award-winning global Dance for PD® program, has taken these results to heart. Since 2001, he and his team have provided dance classes in New York for people living with Parkinson's. Dance for PD has grown worldwide, with classes in more than 450 communities in 28 countries. Fifty-one peer-reviewed scientific studies listed on Dance for PD's website (www.danceforparkinsons.org) provide evidence that underpins the effectiveness and benefits of the Dance for PD teaching practice.

Research shows that the Dance for PD model may relieve debilitating symptoms, aid short-term mobility, significantly improve stability, contribute to social inclusion, improve overall quality of life and self-efficacy, decrease rigidity, and improve facial expression. A longitudinal study published in 2021 suggests that weekly participation in Dance for PD classes over three years may have the potential to slow the progression of motor symptoms in people with PD compared to a nondance cohort.

In Chapter 30, David shares these and other benefits he's observed from experience. His observations may change how you and your loved ones think about living with Parkinson's.

Sometimes the challenges confronting people are not neurology based but psychological. Mental health is a growing concern for all ages. Yes, we know that dance provides social and emotional benefits. But in some cases, dance can provide even more significant benefits as a mental health therapy.

Dance/movement therapy has had surprising results, bringing hope and improvement to patients dealing with anxiety and depression. It also helps people diagnosed with psychotic disorders who are being treated in locked units.

Finally, dancers of all ages must know how to take care of their physical needs. The growing medical specialty of dance medicine builds on the foundation of sports medicine to assist dancers of all levels—from professional ballet dancers to harried working parents who release stress in their weekly hour of social dancing.

Yes, research and case studies are compelling. But human stories make them real.

Chapter 28

⌄

Dementia: Meet Them
Where They Are

We start by telling the story of several courageous ballroom dance professionals. These professionals sought new ways to teach aging dancers who may not remember their own names yet still remember the dance steps they learned long ago.

Despite promising research on how frequent dancing prevents or slows the progress of dementia, there is no real dance training yet available to serve people with dementia. But that hasn't stopped some instructors from developing their own techniques when working with students experiencing memory loss. In some cases, instructors have reached out in partnership with their local Alzheimer's Association to develop new curriculum to teach those with memory loss. These stories are heartwarming.

Over seven years ago, Nathan Daniels started teaching three ballroom dance lessons per week to Anna (not her real name), an older woman he describes yet today as "physically very strong and always immaculately coiffed." She continues to dance the same schedule with Nathan when she isn't traveling. She's missed only a few lessons over that entire time.

After about two years of instruction, Anna began showing signs of memory loss. Nathan noticed that she wouldn't finish conversations, or she'd go in a completely different direction for no apparent reason. Other times, she couldn't remember important details like where she lived.

Through it all, Anna continued to dance and love it, but Nathan noticed "diminishing returns" from their lessons. While Anna's family was aware of her deteriorating health, Nathan was never sure how aware Anna was of it herself, as she was never formally diagnosed with Alzheimer's or another form of dementia.

Nathan had no training in dancing with those living with dementia, so he read up on the subject and went by trial and error. What did he learn?

"The main thing is that you have to meet them where they are and go with that," Nathan said. "You can't put whatever your feelings are or whatever your thoughts are onto them. And you have to try to find what's going to click in."

He found he needed a "whole different skill set" in teaching. This included a different compassion level, different way to talk, and different words to use—or not use.

"You have to be able to pivot all the time, changing what you do, to continue progress forward," Nathan added. "You don't use words like *remember* because they don't, and it makes them feel bad when they can't. It puts them in that negative mind space of 'Oh man, I can't remember that.' So instead of saying 'Remember what I told you about this step?' you just repeat what you said about that step. It's really about compassion and listening and not necessarily wanting a grand result. You want them to have fun and get their money's worth, which just may be having fun."

While Anna can sometimes "recapture" information she already knows, there can't be any new information or input.

"If I try to teach her a new dance, that doesn't work," Nathan said. "It's got to be something she's familiar with, that she can hopefully pull up in the Rolodex in her mind. Sometimes that works, and sometimes it doesn't. She just happens to be very good at following. She does a lot by feel, and not necessarily because her brain is telling her to do this or that. It also depends on the day. Some days are better than others for her retention level. Sometimes I'll say something, and a minute and a half later say the same thing, and she'll act as though I'd never said it. Other times she'll say, 'You just told me that.' So both ends of the spectrum happen, and you don't know which one you're going to get."

How does that feel as a dance teacher?

"The feeling is mostly good," he said. "You know you're doing something they enjoy, and they're getting fun out of it. But you hope you don't do anything that will frustrate them, so it's a little like walking on eggshells. But it's rewarding because you're hopefully adding positivity to their life."

And how's it like for Anna?

"Well, she keeps coming back!" Nathan said. "And music is huge for her. She loves any kind of music. She constantly lets me know that the music is telling her what to do. Well, it's not really 'telling' her to do a heel lead. Sometimes I just go with it, and sometimes the stubborn Nathan comes out and says, 'No, sorry.' Sometimes I catch myself trying to be Nathan the teacher, as opposed to Nathan the compassionate person."

This lovely partnership seems to be working for Nathan and Anna, perhaps because they respectively fall into the traditional leader and follower roles. But what if the student with dementia is a male ballroom dancer who generally is the leader rather than the follower?

Jason (not his real name) has been part of the Minnesota Argentine tango community for twenty years, almost as long as Tango Society organizer and instructor Loisa Donnay (the same instructor who taught Argentine tango to ninety-three-year-old Angela in Chapter 15). Loisa knew Jason as a "very good and dedicated dancer, a good skier, a single guy, and a financial consultant who did well at his job."

Several years ago, Jason fell prey to a financial scam and had an unrelated belligerent run-in with police. Both incidents were clearly out of character. His friends and family could tell that something wasn't right, so they got in touch with Loisa and the tango community. A lawyer from the community also stepped in to help.

Jason went two years without dancing, then another friend suggested that Loisa come to his home to visit him and dance. Loisa started dancing with Jason during the summer of 2020. Despite the two-year break from dancing, it all came back to him.

"He's the leader," Loisa explained. "Somehow, the steps are in his body, in his muscle memory. I don't know what part of his brain they're in. I'm not an expert at this. He takes a woman into his arms, he hears the music, and he starts to move and walk. It's such a learned behavior that it works."

Jason was later relocated to a group home, where Loisa still visits him once a week. She often brings other members of the tango community to dance with him. Even though Jason has little short-term memory, he often remembers Loisa and other friends from his dancing past. He also still recognizes the dance music; he knows which song and orchestra is which. All that is still a very big part of his memory.

It's remarkable, even if he isn't able to learn new steps.

"Sometimes the only thing I can do is correct some steps, remind him why that step didn't work, and maybe show how he could do it this way," Loisa said. "I don't try to teach him anything new. He's not interested in that. He's interested in just playing with the music and dancing whenever or whatever he can."

Jason's story is a beacon of hope for all dancers.

"What I'm saying here is that dance is a hobby that stays with you through thick and thin," Loisa said. "When all other abilities go away, you might still be able to dance. And there is the wonderful advantage of dance community. People who you know as honest will remember you, will surround you, will come to your aid, and will have expertise. There's an honesty there that you may not find if you just googled for an attorney, for example. You're reaching out to your friends and community, who of course have a reputation. You have volunteers who are able to talk and visit with you, help you out, and be part of your life at your tougher moments."

In addition to the memory issues, Jason also has aphasia, a brain condition that makes it difficult to speak effectively. What is it like to teach Jason under these circumstances?

"He's always at the door, waiting for me to come," Loisa replied. "It's quite rewarding. And it's still nice to dance with him, even though it's getting harder and harder to communicate with him. I'm just going over there and brightening his day a little bit. That's really my scope here. I have no training for this, so I don't know if I'm helping in a clinical way. All I know is I'm going over there and he's happy to see me. He's happy to see anyone I bring along. I do feel I'm improving his quality of life. There's a benefit I'm giving him."

Having known Jason before and after his conditions set in, Loisa was surprised by an unexpected change in his personality.

"Jason is a very proud man, proud of his accomplishments, his skiing, his travel," she said. "That part of his personality has changed. He's more humble now than he was. It is really different to deal with him."

Though Loisa and Jason are still dancing once a week, he's less agile these days. That's likely in part because he and the other residents in his new care home have little chance for exercise. But Loisa believes that dancing has helped his mobility.

"His reaction as soon as I turn on the music is still wonderful to see," Loisa said. "He visibly brightens and moves with the rhythm. He reaches for anyone around him to dance, to the delight of his caregivers. One of his caregivers was even inspired to start dance lessons!"

The individual partnerships between Nathan and Anna and Loisa and Jason show how productive, joyful, and beneficial it can be to dance with people living with memory issues. The dance world needs to scale up these efforts and develop classes that specifically serve elder adults or those with early symptoms of dementia. That said, I'm aware of only a few entrepreneurial dance instructors who were working pre-pandemic to do such a thing. I give each of these instructors great credit.

One such effort in Minnesota was led by Beyond Ballroom Dance Company and its cofounder Deanne Michael, in collaboration with the Alzheimer's Association in Minnesota. As Deanne's former dance partner, Nathan Daniels was a teacher for that pilot class.

Nathan recalled that there were about seven or eight participants, mainly people living with dementia. They danced together as partners. In one case, a woman living with dementia attended in her wheelchair and danced with her husband, her caretaker.

Working one-on-one is different from working with a group class. The challenge in a group class is that it changes every time. Different people might attend, and they might be at different levels of dementia.

"You have to feel the tenor of the room," Nathan said.

How do you measure success in such a changing group situation?

"What you're trying to do is help them have fun, laugh, and move their body," Nathan explained. "What I think they wanted was to get out of their normal surroundings, have a sense of community, touch each other, and be able to move and use their brain."

Unfortunately, the pilot class was short lived, as interest from the local Alzheimer's Association waned.

A similar class was started in New York City. In 2019, Esther Frances, a ballroom dance professional and then manager and instructor at an Arthur Murray Dance Studio in Manhattan, stepped up. She knew the effects of Alzheimer's firsthand, as she'd watched family members live with it.

"I've seen how quickly people can decline if they don't take action," she said. "People sometimes think 'action' means taking medicine or seeing a doctor. But it means being more active and taking care of yourself and doing something like dancing, which can have so many different benefits. I wanted to bring that to more people."

Esther partnered with an early-stage social engagement program offered by the local Alzheimer's Association chapter. Together, they created a pilot program at her studio that ran two sessions per week for five weeks. It wasn't easy, though. Esther booked group classes, engaged four or five volunteer staff, and learned new ways to teach, all without funding or compensation.

The Alzheimer's Association trained the instructors before the classes started. However, the instructors soon found that the goal was not to teach basic ballroom dance. Rather, the classes were more movement based and repetitive. Still, the students did learn formal dances. They started with the basic merengue and moved to Argentine tango. They then performed at the prescheduled showcases for all students at the studio.

Esther explained that teaching people with memory loss is different in three ways from teaching other students.

First, people with Alzheimer's experience problems with balance. This means multiple staff professionals are needed to teach the class and physically help students balance as they learn the steps. Students began by marching side to side to become more aware of their bodies and posture.

"You help them balance," Esther recalled. "And depending on their state of Alzheimer's, they have different levels of balance on their standing leg. But by the end, they actually could do basic steps."

Second, multiple approaches are needed. Learning to music is "super helpful" for some students but not all.

"We had to find ways that are safe for everybody," Esther said. "You have to play music, you have to use numbers, you have to use vocals. Most respond a lot better with touch."

And that brings us to the third point: Touch is key when working with people with Alzheimer's.

"You have to help them feel where to go," Esther said. "You can tell them what a backstep is, but you may need to help people move through it. You have to physically do that."

One of the best parts of the program was that caregivers, too, saw benefits when they joined in the fun with their partners.

"The caregivers had such an amazing time," Esther said. "It was great for them to have a mental break, where they could just have fun with each other. A break from caregiving is so important. People forget that," she added.

And the dancers?

"They loved it," she said. "They loved the music, the movement, and the dancing. They loved the whole activity—getting dressed, coming to the studio, getting dressed for a show, getting a pair of dance shoes, doing makeup and hair, and doing the performance."

As the program played out, Esther observed actual evidence of improvement.

"I did see the difference," said Esther. "You might have somebody at the beginning of the class who could barely stand on their two feet, and then a couple weeks later, they're doing a tango basic. I would say that's a pretty big success. But you have to maintain it."

Unfortunately, the program didn't continue once the pandemic hit. Esther moved to Florida and became an independent instructor. But even now, in a post-pandemic world, there are still barriers.

"There's a lack of funding for these programs," Esther said. "Our project was volunteer based, and the volunteers had to be certified to work with people with Alzheimer's. And on their end, the Alzheimer's Association didn't have enough staff or caregivers to bring the patients to the studio."

How do we begin to scale up dance programming so more seniors with dementia can be served?

We need many more Esthers, Deannes, Nathans, and Loisas willing to give their gifts and talents to people living with dementia. They are out there, I know. Many of my dance teacher friends and even amateur dancers tell me they want to help.

But the effort also needs funding for staffing and training. It takes a solid infrastructure to train local teachers and educate health care leaders around the country about the great need and clear results of the research.

Enter ballroom professional Wayne Eng, founder and chief executive officer of Dance Vision (an online producer of ballroom dance education materials) and chairman of the prestigious Emerald Ball Dancesport Championship in Los

Angeles. In 2018 Wayne and his wife, Donna, created the Dance Vision Foundation, a nonprofit allowing them to give back to the dance community by providing the benefits of dance to those who couldn't afford it.

And when they personally observed the positive effects dance had on a dear friend and employee who suffered from bipolar disorder and other mental health issues, they found their mission. The couple geared their dance activities toward mental wellness and brain health. They chose to start with older adults, addressing Alzheimer's, dementia, Parkinson's, and other conditions that could benefit from the brain-and-body coordination of ballroom dance. Eventually, they want to expand their mental wellness focus to other generations, as people of all ages can benefit from dance.

In late 2023, Wayne found an ally in ballroom dance judge Maria Hansen, an accomplished competitive dancer and thirty-eight-year ballroom dance teacher. Maria had been a nursing student before she turned to dance, and her interest in biology, biomechanics, health, and wellness has never waned. After she retired from competitive dance, she studied kinesiology because she wanted to learn about movement from a more scientific perspective. And when Wayne asked Maria to be part of the Dance Vision Foundation, she focused first on research and creating pilot classes.

Maria knew she was on the right path during the very first class she tested in Carmel, California. She met a man with the difficult diagnosis of Lewy body dementia. His wife was worried about him joining the class, but Maria suggested he might just enjoy the music.

"About the third song in, he decided he wanted to get up and dance with his wife," Maria recalled. "She was in shock because he never liked to get out of his chair. So they swayed back and forth in the back of the room. He hugged her and kissed her and then sat back down, joining the class with movements in his chair. It was a really special moment for them and also for me. I felt like what I was doing was being validated."

Maria knew from her research that music memories are stored in a different part of the brain—the last part of the brain that is affected by Alzheimer's.

"That's why the generational music we choose is so important," Maria added. "It activates every region of the brain."

Maria has also worked with a physical therapist in Seattle to start an ongoing class in a retirement center. Some people can stand, and some are in wheelchairs.

"There was one lady who was pretty nonresponsive," Maria said. "She was hunched over in her chair and didn't make eye contact when I tried to introduce myself. But about halfway into the first song, she made eye contact with me. Then she started bouncing up and down in her chair, trying to copy my arm movements. It was like a light had lit inside her, and she smiled the most beautiful smile I've ever seen. It could light up New York! Then in the middle of the class, she wanted to stand up. So the physical therapist brought her a ballet barre, and we helped her stand and hold the barre, joining the rest of the class. It was a forty-five-minute class, but all the participants wanted to keep going, so I did another forty-five minutes. And this woman still wanted to stay after that. It was beautiful to see someone come to life that way."

As Maria and her colleagues move beyond the testing phase with their pilot classes, the foundation's intention is to develop an outreach program. They want to create classes in retirement homes, assisted-living facilities, senior community centers, and eventually hospital systems. They will train and pay teachers, though many people want to volunteer as well. And the good news is, these volunteers don't have to be dance teachers.

"They just have to be people who care," Maria said. "The biggest things are enthusiasm, compassion, and empathy for what we're doing and the people we're doing it for. The routines aren't difficult to do. The way I choreograph the music makes it very simple to teach, learn, and do."

The goal is to have the choreography routines explained in writing and in video on a private YouTube channel so people can easily learn how to lead classes. The routines would be changed up periodically to keep things fresh.

As Maria looks to the long-term future, she's passionate about creating classes for other generations, such as Generation X and Millennials, to address anxiety, stress, and mental well-being.

"Studies show that dancing is actually more effective than drugs in combating anxiety and stress," she said. "Every generation has issues. The sad thing is that the Zoomers, the youngest generation, has the highest suicide rate of all. They're the generation that has grown up on social media, and that's creating a lot of problems for them."

Kudos to the Dance Vision Foundation and all the dance professionals leading the way both pre- and post-pandemic to bring benefits of partner dance to boomers and elder adults living with Alzheimer's and dementia. The possibilities are endless. The vision is real. The need is huge.

But a few individuals and a single foundation can only do so much. While other organizations are stepping up, the efforts are fragmented and uncoordinated across the country.

That's why we need a Call to Action. Stay tuned for more in Part VI.

Chapter 29

Taking On Parkinson's
Disease Together

"I think it's Parkinson's," the general practice physician told Michael Finney over six years ago. "If it is, we're gonna deal with it."

Michael, then fifty-eight, presented a tremor in his right hand, had recently fallen off a ladder, and had a family history of essential tremors.

"I felt the initial 'Oh my God—my life is over,'" Michael recalled. "But in reality, I had worked with people with Parkinson's for most of my career. I knew there were things you could do to improve your quality of life. It was a question of knuckling down and doing it."

And he did. When first diagnosed, Michael was rated a nine on a scale measuring Parkinson's impairment. Six years later, he was a four.

"I've actually been decreasing the degree of impairment over the course," he said. "It's not like it goes into remission or anything. But a lot of the functional balance training and functional strength training translates into a much better quality of life."

Michael still works around the world, managing the design and production of visitor experiences ranging from museum attractions to *The Making of Harry Potter* for Warner Bros.

Studio Tour London. He did cut back on physical site inspections, though, so he could focus more on the teaching side, which he loves.

"It probably isn't a good idea for me to be climbing up on high steel installations anymore, anyway," he said with a laugh.

Michael sees the advantage of putting someone with a later-life issue, such as Parkinson's disease, in front of younger learners.

"You can have PD *and* you can be doing a very cool thing with your life. That's one of the reasons why I don't hide my diagnosis," he said.

Michael isn't managing this alone. He's a strong advocate for the Struthers Parkinson's Center in Golden Valley, Minnesota. Struthers provided him a holistic approach to dealing with Parkinson's in mind, body, and spirit for over four years.

And he is an unabashed admirer of his wife, Linda Muir, a well-known ballet teacher in the Twin Cities. Linda has danced ballet and modern dance for sixty of her sixty-four years, has performed in dance companies throughout the country, and has been teaching children at dance studios since she moved to Minnesota twenty-four years ago.

As a professionally trained dancer, Linda was eligible to enroll in the New York–based Mark Morris Dance Group's Dance for PD program. This training combined with her years of professional dance experience and her collaboration with physical and music therapists have made her a powerful volunteer teacher for Struthers—and for Michael.

Perhaps most unusual about this couple is that they *both* understand, at a professional level, the value of connecting art and science. Linda has been interested in the science of the brain for years.

"We must open our minds to what the sciences can offer our art form," she said. "Dance is taught through oral history, passed down from generation to generation. How we do things is not necessarily scientifically based, but science can inform a great deal. Because of my interest on both sides, I see how the two can inform each other. I understand how dance can change the neurological pathways of the brain, replacing those pathways closed off because of Parkinson's disease. I understand from the science that new pathways can be created. And the way to creating those pathways is new movement learning. Any new experience, if it can be related to the life of the person with Parkinson's, will both enrich their spirit and support the development of the plasticity of their mind, their brain. It's a complex world that comes down to something simple."

Linda is working with Michael's physical therapist and music therapist at Struthers. Sometimes it's three-on-one when working with Michael.

"I kind of straddle the two worlds," Linda said. "I understand movement to music, and I understand how to communicate that to participants. That's what I do as a teacher. And I understand what a physical therapist is trying to do because I understand anatomy and kinesiology and how our bodies work. They accept my expertise, and we learn together. It's a good working relationship."

Linda believes she's learned as much from that interaction as from the Mark Morris course.

Michael also straddles both worlds. "I'm the answer to what you do for a career when you have a degree in theater and in engineering," he said.

His first love was theater, but engineering was always a viable career for him because his father was an engineer. In college, then, he started in theater but got to a point where he wanted to build new structures and buildings. So he built a degree program that let him pursue both. At one point, his class schedule included Ballet, Theatre History, Strength of Materials, and Engineering Management.

"You sprain your brain that way," he said.

Michael danced ballet and modern dance during college, and he even did some ballroom when "thrown into" musicals that needed another man.

"My physical therapist recently asked me, 'Why do you point your foot every time it comes off the floor? That must be more challenging.' I don't think about it. I was taught when your foot leaves the floor, it points."

Today, Michael manages large projects for his entertainment design firm, putting him squarely between the creative, artistic side and the engineering, construction side.

"The running joke is that I'm the one who translates," he said. "I speak both languages, artistic and technical."

Kind of like Linda.

Linda credits Michael's improvement to movement and the related therapies she and his therapists have developed since other factors such as medications have not changed. But she also credits Michael himself.

"He is by nature an optimistic person," she said. "And from day one, he's been engaged in the physical activity he needs to do. If he doesn't get something right away, he insists on continuing it until he gets it. He's very invested in doing everything that he can do to stave off symptoms for as long as possible. That is invaluable. Period. Attitude!"

During the COVID pandemic, Linda and Michael worked in their home studio space.

"We have mirrors, which are an important component for people with Parkinson's to see," Linda explained. "They can often perceive that they're not using opposite limbs, for instance, when they watch. Their proprioception doesn't give them the feedback from inside their body. So the fact that we have full mirrors, where he can observe himself, is important. And often, if he's not getting something, he can get it from following me. I'll physically do with him what I'm asking him to do."

Linda continued, "I don't really dance with him. I create movement exercises that work on coordination, balance, range of motion, and also cognition. I've learned a lot from the physical therapist here at Struthers. We do an exercise with a walking stick, where he twists and does relevés, and we might have him say a different woman's name each time starting with C, like *Carol*. So now not only is he having to *learn* a physical sequence and actually *do* a physical sequence, but he also has to put a cognitive aspect to it."

Michael sees it this way: "It's a lot of alignment, a lot of balance transitional work. Moving from static position to static position dynamically has been incredibly good. My balance is such that I was slipping on ice in winter yet able to catch myself before I fell—it's really good. Both Linda and my physical therapist have been doing a lot of work with me by giving me cognitive challenges to perform while I'm doing balance-based exercise. They especially focus on diagonal and crossbody, which helps your speed of motion, helps your proprioception. That's one of the things I lost when PD came on. I was losing track of where my body was in space. Stupid things—like bumping my hip on the kitchen table, reaching for something and missing it by six inches. Doing a lot of this exercise has helped that tremendously."

Now that Michael is rated as a four on the impairment scale, what are his current symptoms?

"I have vocal stuff occasionally. I can't speak for hours at a time, like I used to—which may be good," he joked. "I'm still dealing with tremor. But I don't have to be as consciously aware of my balance as when I was first diagnosed. The big thing is tremor and speed of movement. Speed of movement is not coming back. I don't move as fast as I did previously, especially if I'm thinking about moving fast. But if I'm just letting the body do its thing, I do OK. One of the big issues with Parkinson's is falls. I haven't had a fall."

So what is it like to work with your wife as teacher?

Michael laughed. "Well, she's probably the best ballet teacher I've ever worked with. She has extraordinary ability to teach motion. The great thing is that she obviously knows how I move. The challenge for her—or for both of us—is that she's my wife, and she hates to see me struggle with something. But the good thing is that because of her professional experience, she'll let me struggle with it until I get it. I get a little bull-headed about this—'I will get this right.' If I do an exercise, I don't count the movements I do wrong. That's the dancer background. It's like you don't repeat and learn the wrong movement. The other good thing? I've got a resource that I can look at in the morning and ask, 'Am I moving funny?' And she will tell me."

For Linda, it's all about trust.

"There's a trust that I'm trying to do what is best and beneficial for him, that I have expertise to back that up, and that there will be continuing communication. 'Is this too much for you?' or 'Linda, this is too complicated—we need to step back a bit.' That's because his cognition is very good at this time. It's that idea of trust and, of course, love and understanding."

As to the future?

"Cognitively, Michael is really with it," Linda said. "For that, I'm grateful. One of my goals is to keep him doing the work he loves for as long as we can make that happen. For me, one way I manage this whole thing is to say 'What's in front of me today?' and not concern myself with what will happen. I don't have control of that. We have control of taking our meds, doing our exercise, having a fulfilling life as well as we can, for today. Period."

Michael is looking further out. Professionally, he's making some adjustments, such as choosing not to temporarily relocate to Japan for a project. He packs lighter in his carry-on suitcase. He provides more time for sleep after travel. He carries a motion tracker app on his phone that's basically a fall alert that calls Linda or 911 if it receives no movement response.

For Michael, dance movement is working.

"It's given me control of how I deal with my motion challenges," he said. "It's given me a toolbox. It's hardwired some coping skills to a degree that would not be possible with just regular exercise. It keeps me interested because there's an endless variety of options for how to teach movement, balance, and application of strength. It gives me community, which I think is incredibly valuable. I'm doing things I've never done before. Some things I'm doing I thought I stopped doing in my twenties. Apparently not."

Michael is just one person of many around the globe who has benefited from a trained teaching artist from Dance for PD. Thankfully, there are hundreds of Lindas.

We go next to New York City, home of Dance for PD and its cofounder, David Leventhal.

Chapter 30

⌄

There Are No Patients.
There Are Only Dancers.

The dancers (nearly all older adults) on the stage of the famous Mark Morris Dance Center in New York City form a large circle, holding hands, gliding back and forth to the classical music of Mozart. The scene is reminiscent of a minuet. The group of about twenty dancers "scallop" as they weave through the circle to hold hands with new partners.

Later, all the dancers are seated, using their arms and legs to improvise small movements, then using their entire bodies to stretch in all directions, opening their bodies and their hearts to the audience, the community, and the world.

Soon, Manny and Joy come out to an empty stage. Manny is seated stage left in a tux with a loose bow tie hanging around his neck. Joy comes from the right in a slimming, long red gown.

As the waltz music begins, they slowly come together, as if making up after a fight. They elegantly dance together in waltz frame, then dance separately, seemingly conflicted as to whether they want to be together again.

Near the end, Cyndy, another dancer, does an exquisite solo performance, turning, twisting, bending, reaching to the sky, using every limb to its fullest extension.

The audience in this premiere dance theater is mesmerized. They cheer wildly after each segment in the hour-long show. For good reason.

Nearly all the dancers on stage are living with Parkinson's disease.

Some are newly diagnosed. Others have been diagnosed for twenty-plus years. All of them attended dance classes for a full year through Dance for PD with David Leventhal, one of the program's founding teachers and formerly a lead dancer with the Mark Morris Dance Group.

"It's not like the experience of dance is in any way a cure," David said. "But it transports the dancers to a completely different level. In that state of flow and fluidity, Parkinson's is nowhere in the room. It's miles away."

As class member Reggie said, "There are no patients. There are only dancers."

This is the story of a project that took place in 2011, as told in the award-winning documentary *Capturing Grace*, directed by David Iverson and filmed in collaboration with the Brooklyn Parkinson Group, the Mark Morris Dance Group, and Dance for PD.

In the film, we meet Cyndy, the solo dancer diagnosed with Parkinson's twenty-four years prior.

"Sometimes I can't walk, but I can dance," she says.

At home, she shows a tremor in her hand; she shuffles as she walks in short, halting steps. She presents characteristically jerky, unpredictable movements in her torso and arms.

Then she dances. The tremor is gone. Her arms are outstretched as she sways them side to side. She lightly glides across the living room floor, almost sweeping and sliding her feet around the room. There is no jerkiness, just fluidity and elegance. Her joy is unmistakable.

On performance day, Cyndy reads her personal note from David: "When you dance, you bring the whole world in and reveal your whole self. Enjoy today."

Joy tells us, "Dance works against the natural inclination that Parkinson's has to constrict and hunch over. Dance straightens you up and extends your arms."

David gave Joy a note as well: "You take light and turn it into movement. The photosynthesis of sorts. You dance with clarity and honesty."

And in Manny's note, David wrote: "You dance with your heart and soul. And share so much of yourself with all of us. Enjoy today, savor it."

The Mark Morris Dance Group first offered classes for people living with Parkinson's in 2001. Today, the award-winning Dance for PD initiative is global. They offer a research-backed program for people with Parkinson's and their families, with classes online, in New York City, and through a network of partners and affiliates in more than 450 communities in 28 countries. In New York City, classes are offered in English, Spanish, and Mandarin.

The classes are transformative for people with PD. In fact, David often sees dramatic transformation during a one-hour class.

"Dance seems to fit Parkinson's like a glove," he began. "Parkinson's is a disease of subtraction. So over time, things get taken away. Strengths or skills you used to have, particularly the 'automatic' ones, are more difficult to access. But the thing is, Parkinson's is more than just a movement disorder. It's a quality-of-life condition—it affects all aspects of an individual's life. So it's also about self-esteem, confidence, sense of connection to others, self-identity, and self-efficacy, which is the feeling that you have the power to do something. It also affects mood. More than 50 percent of people with Parkinson's are living with some degree of depression. It creates anxiety. All these elements percolate through every component of somebody's life. What's remarkable is that dance has a way of addressing each of those things through this art form, but it does it almost unconsciously."

Dance for PD includes all styles of dance.

"We are nondenominational in terms of dance," David explained. "Each teacher teaches what they know—whether you are a salsa expert or traditional Chinese dance teacher. It's not the style that makes this program effective; it's the fact that dance of whatever form shares a common DNA. It's like humans. Though we may look and sound a bit different, depending on our background, we share 99.9 percent of our DNA. Dance is like that too. When you look at the fundamentals of any dance technique from the motor-skill level, from the imaginative level, from the music and storytelling levels, we share it all. The DNA is there. It's that DNA that's so powerful for people with Parkinson's."

So what exactly is that DNA?

"We see a couple things happen," David said. "First is fluidity of movement. The sense of one movement leading into the next—which is like the way we speak, as opposed to stopping at every word. Parkinson's movement is absence of flow. So one of the first things I see as we start to piece movement phrases together is that a sense of flow comes back into the body. People are thinking about how to create a movement sentence that has a flow to it."

Along with that comes a focus on movement quality.

"People with Parkinson's—and even the general public—are focused on the steps," David said. "'Do I go right? Do I go front or back? Which leg is it?' Our classes focus on the *how*. It doesn't matter whether you go left or right but *how* you are stepping. Are you stepping through water? Are you escaping from something? Are you reaching to someone you love? What is the motivation behind your movement? When you do that, you start to engage the imagination, and you start to engage the emotions behind the movement. It's like an actor."

David uses the imagination in service of story.

"That part of the brain is very much active and is able to generate or spark movement even though the mechanics of that movement may be cumbersome," he said. "And by doing that, we see people accessing movement that they had trouble accessing before."

This is how we tell a story through dance. Take a Broadway show like *West Side Story* for example.

"We see the movements become strong, powerful, and rhythmic," David said. "They're able to travel through space as a Shark or a Jet because they're fully invested in the story they're trying to tell with their bodies."

And what is David's vision for the future?

"The keywords for us are *access* and *inclusion*. How do we make this program available to as many people as we can? And once available, how do we make sure they have a sense of belonging in that experience?"

With classes available online and in-person across the globe, David focuses on making the classes culturally responsive to those in each room. For example, when working with the Hmong community, the music and movement should reflect Hmong cultural traditions. To that end, Dance for PD is offering training for teachers around the world. That training features the core structure and approach of the program, but it allows flexibility for the content to be locally created and tailored.

David also wants to see the program offered as a standard health intervention throughout the dance community, such as in dance studios and companies and in university dance programs. And he wants to see dance embedded in standard clinical care, with access as common as physical therapy.

That's already starting. Since the pandemic, many people have reached out to Dance for PD directly.

"They've flat-out called us and asked us to start a program in their communities," David said. "They're not people with Parkinson's. They're neurologists. They're medical and health care centers telling us, 'We want this.' And we're seeing an increase in assisted-living facilities asking for this program."

Even a large national health insurer requested David and the Mark Morris team to adapt the Dance for PD model to a general curriculum for the retiree groups within their Medicare Advantage programs.

And more and more dance professionals and volunteers are stepping up to help.

These are breakthroughs. The tools are here. The need is great.

The key is scale. We must find ways to scale up proven effective programming that brings dance and arts into health care. There are many successful initiatives across the country. Dance for PD is just one. But somehow David and his team have grown Dance for PD to 450 sites around the world. How did they do that? What new and innovative strategies are helping them to grow? What can other leaders in the arts and health space learn from their success?

As David told his dancers before going onstage in New York, "You know what to do. It's all there."

And perhaps it is. We go there next.

Chapter 31

⌣

Scaling Up Dance for PD®

Scaling up any new initiative takes enormous time, resources, and "boots on the ground," especially when introducing something into a very large and complex national health care system. But once there is a breakthrough, the doors open for others to follow.

Dance for PD has created breakthroughs in two ways: 1) partnering with a large US Medicare Advantage program for financial support; and 2) scaling up its training model to reach more dance teachers and volunteers around the globe.

This is a big deal.

Bringing National Medicare Advantage Programs to the Table

As I talked with physicians and scientists across the country to research this book, the reaction was consistent when I told them that a national health care insurer was purchasing dance services from Dance for PD. It was: "Wow! Really?"

Yes, really. It was in May of 2022 that David was contacted by a representative of the insurer to learn more about dance for health programming. They were interested in more than a subset population of those living with Parkinson's. So David and the Mark Morris Dance Group offered a "Move and Flow" program geared for a more general senior elder population. That seemed to fit. A pilot online program was initiated in fall 2022 to a small group of members. The response from members and clients was strong, so the insurer rolled out the initiative to all its retiree groups on January 1, 2023. (The insurer is not named to ensure privacy for its members.)

"This is a health insurance company saying 'We want to promote health through engagement in dance and other art forms,'" said David. "It's a huge shift from wondering whether dance might ever be covered by insurance to where we're seeing insurance companies actually engaging dance organizations to offer dance programming geared towards healthy living. That's very exciting."

David wants to see every insurance company and medical center do this, which also sends the message that dance classes are valuable and offer benefits to their members. This strategy is different from the popular SilverSneakers program. "This approach incentivizes the physical and social emotional benefits of dance, rather than pays each individual to do it. It is the bulk model: Let's pay for the programming and let people come to it," said David. "It's a drop in the bucket in terms of paying for health benefits."

Monthly virtual classes are scheduled by the insurer well in advance, usually on the same day and time each month. The classes are offered to members of all their retiree groups, and the insurer is invoiced for each class after it occurs. Between three hundred and one thousand members typically register for the classes, with about 35 to 40 percent or more signing on and attending.

It didn't take long for the insurer to start conducting occasional pilot in-person dance classes in a few dance studios around the country. They work with their interested customers to bring the program to a location where large numbers of members reside. David connects them with a local dance studio and instructor. A member of their team travels to the site to provide remarks at the one-time event and greet the members.

David then invoices the insurer after the event for all related costs, including fees for the studio and the instructor.

Members report that they love both the virtual and in-person events. Members say they want more—they want to dance more than once a month. Participants sometimes share that the program helps with a shoulder or knee problem. They like the option to stand or sit for the class. And when they are on camera, people are seen dancing around the living room with their partner. Caregivers sometimes help them to participate. Some sit in a recliner and move their arms to dance. Sometimes they just watch and love the social connection.

This feedback led to offering a wide variety of video on-demand classes that members could access on their own, including many different forms of dance. The offerings are periodically updated. Dance for PD manages access to the videos through a contract similar to a limited licensing agreement.

Participation in this program is currently limited by the insurer to groups that consist primarily of retirees. Most of these members are sixty-five-plus years of age. Individual members of the health plan or members of active employee plans are not yet eligible. But this is a good start.

Dance for PD is on to something big in partnering with this health care provider. Kudos to them both. Which Medicare Advantage program will be next to bring dance for health to its members? What other medical institutions will step up in the same way and bring programming to their patients and even their health care employees?

Older adults can't wait.

Dance Teacher: "One of the Best Things I've Done with My Life"

You are not affiliated with a large health care organization or insurance company. You are just one dancer, a teacher, or dance ally, who wants to help bring dance for health to your community. How can you help? Consider becoming a Dance for PD teaching artist or volunteer like Jessica, Libby, and Linda, below. They started years ago by traveling to small training classes primarily in New York City. But here's the breakthrough. If this is of interest to you, Dance for PD has found an easier way to scale up training of teaching artists and volunteers. Stay tuned.

Jessica Roeder, a modern dance and writing teacher from Duluth, Minnesota, was an early trainee. Over thirteen years ago Jessica saw a video email about the international award-winning Dance for PD initiative through the Mark Morris Dance Group, one of her favorite dance companies. Tears came to her eyes—joyful tears. It was Christmas Eve. She signed up online that very night to volunteer if this was happening in Minnesota. Within a half hour of her hitting "Send," David Leventhal responded. "It's not happening in Minnesota yet. Would you be interested in training to teach?"

Jessica obtained a grant through the Arrowhead Regional Arts Council and headed to Brooklyn, New York, to the Mark Morris Dance Center. "I was really nervous, but I felt so at home there. David is a very kind person—he is warm, he remembers people. I can't say enough about him as a teacher. It's amazing because he is such a wonderful dancer, and he also has this gift for teaching."

Somehow it was meant to be. At the end of the training, Jessica's Dance for PD class was joined by people with Parkinson's. David paired up people to massage each other's hands. "So here is this man with Parkinson's from Manhattan, I'm massaging his hands, and he tells me he is from Duluth, Minnesota!" recalled Jessica.

She returned home to start a class. At a local wedding, she met Joan Setterlund, a woman with Parkinson's who wanted to participate and help. Together, Joan and Jessica got the word out and found accessible space at the newly built Unitarian Universalist Church in Duluth. There was no start-up funding, but it didn't matter. "Just start the class because you are going to love doing it," a friend who started the class in Chicago told

Jessica. "Just get it started and worry about the rest later." The seventy-five-minute classes started once a week. "I think that was great advice," said Jessica.

Over thirteen years later, Joan Setterlund still attends the weekly dance classes, now an hour long. Classes are currently six to eight students, though numbers were in the high teens to low twenties pre-pandemic. "Usually when people dedicate to it, they stay and don't miss a whole lot of classes," said Jessica. But sadly they lose members due to progression of illness.

Jessica, now in her mid-fifties, continues to volunteer her time teaching the class. Her husband David Caligiuri has been the volunteer class assistant from the start, providing general support to Jessica and participants, constructing and maintaining portable barres, handling the music during class, and demonstrating dance moves for seated attendees.

There is a suggested donation of $3 per person or $5 for a family group to (partially) cover expenses. No one is turned away if they can't pay.

"It's one of my favorite hours of the week every week," said Jessica. "There's a lot of preparation that goes into it, but it is always worth it. No matter how many people attend, there's a joy of connection and dancing. I love dancing whenever I do it, but this class is special. They are dancers. It's one of the best things I've done in my life, one of the things that has meant the most to me. You can't beat it, really. I will continue this as long as I'm around, and as long as people still keep coming."

Jessica loves the community that forms with it. "Everyone supports each other so beautifully, and they celebrate each other too. It's something they often look forward to; it's something that people as a couple or with their children can do together every week that is not a doctor's appointment. This is different; this is just for fun." Remarkably, she found her dancers willing to explore all styles of dance and "jump into" improvisations.

Duluth is just one of the 450-plus sites around the world of the global program Dance for PD. While Jessica teaches unpaid in Duluth, that kind of long-term volunteer commitment is very unusual. Most programs are financially supported by organizations and institutions. Jessica would love to have that institutional support. Currently she is also responsible for recruiting participants, marketing, responding to inquiries, maintaining the website, and sending weekly emails—all the maintenance that goes with operating a quality program. And though she receives requests to assist people with other neuro diseases such as MS and dementia, she simply cannot meet the need.

We need to change that. We need more institutional support and funding for Dance for PD across the nation. Dance for PD is the core curriculum geared for people living with Parkinson's, different from the more general senior curriculum sought by the health insurer above.

One form of that support occurred in the mid-2000s at Bethesda Hospital in St. Paul. Libby Lincoln of Minneapolis taught that weekly class. Libby was an in-house lawyer in Minneapolis for almost thirty years. She also was a trained ballet and jazz dancer who taught jazz dance during law school and her first several years of law practice to maintain her "sanity," she says. While attending a conference in San Francisco, her husband handed her a newspaper article about David Leventhal and Dance for PD. Libby's mother was living with Parkinson's, so Libby was familiar with her symptoms and movement issues.

"I called David, and he said, 'We're doing a workshop in New York, come on out.'" She did. Bethesda had contacted David about starting a program, so the match was made.

"It was wonderful," recalled Libby. "We had everyone from young and recently diagnosed to people in wheelchairs. You just adapt what the movement is to fit what everybody is able to do. We did tap routines, we did Broadway complete with top hats, and we had a flamenco teacher come in." The class, supported by Bethesda as part of their Neurology and Parkinson's program, ranged from two to twenty people per week and caregivers were often involved.

"I think one of the biggest things was the camaraderie," said Libby. "The sense of support, the laughter. Everyone was able to appreciate and laugh at the challenges we faced. We were not looking at this as therapy—we taught it as a dance class."

The program lasted about two years at Bethesda, when they lost the person administering the program. Libby didn't have the bandwidth during her law practice to take on the administrative details. "I just wanted to teach," she said. The program ended, and in 2020, Bethesda Hospital closed. But Libby is still involved as an advocate for her husband, who currently is living with Parkinson's, and as a member of the Patient Advisory Board at Struthers Parkinson's Center (Struthers) in Golden Valley.

Struthers is also the center where Linda Muir, whom you met earlier in this Part V, conducted a series of thirty-minute Zoom classes for people living with Parkinson's during the pandemic years. As Linda advocated for her husband who was diagnosed with Parkinson's, she used her Dance for PD training to voluntarily create her own programming at Struthers.

I watched Linda demonstrate her dance routine with elegant stretches and rhythmic dance movements as Frank Sinatra crooned "Fly Me to the Moon." I could barely resist the impulse to follow her every move or dance my arms, body, and hips. Linda was sitting in a chair, but somehow she was engaging every part of her body, even her feet and legs. And her joy was unmistakable.

Movement is important. But the cognitive part of dance is key.

"As a dancer, you learn a sequence of movements like sentences, and those sentences create a paragraph and then a story," said Linda. "When pedaling a bike you might consider how high you are rotating the pedals, but the reality is you are doing a very high repetition of one action. In dance you are sequencing different kinds of motions and coordinating your arms and legs and your facings, and that supports your cognition.

"There is the concept of brain dance. These [exercises] go through all the developmental phases that we do as a child to build our neurological pathways for learning. Simple things as crossing your limbs across your body or opening and expanding your body and becoming small help rebuild neurological pathways that may have diminished with Parkinson's."

Dance also helps people with Parkinson's with knowledge of their body in space. People with Parkinson's lose the ability to understand where they are in space. Their proprioception is diminished.

Continued Linda, "They may not understand that they are moving very slowly or very small, or which arm they are using. What dance does is free them from being concerned about the specifics and to simply follow along. Because my motion is reflected to them, they can mirror that motion. It becomes easier for them to experience the expansive movement because they are following somebody who is moving expansively."

While Linda continues to support her husband in his efforts to stave off progression of the disease, she has ended her voluntary Zoom classes at Struthers to return to her primary purpose of teaching ballet full time and guiding young dancers.

These three teachers illustrate that well-trained dance teacher artists can make a big impact on individual and community health. It's the power of one plus one plus one.

Jessica, Libby, and Linda are just three of about 1,750 dance teachers who had been trained by Dance for PD through 2024. About 800 teachers are like Jessica, actively teaching the regular curriculum in about 450 sites around the globe. Others offer their expertise outside the formal curriculum structure, as Linda did, often adapting what they've learned to different settings. That works too. *All* are needed to meet the growing demand in community.

According to the Parkinson's Foundation, nearly one million people in the United States were living with Parkinson's disease in 2024; this is expected to rise to 1.2 million by 2030. Minnesota is one of the highest incidence states per capita, with approximately 13,400 people living with Parkinson's. Yet Duluth is the only location in the state where a regular weekly class exists. Minnesota is not alone in this public health service challenge.

There are many more dance teaching artists who may want to bring this special purpose to their lives. Teaching artists, says David, "are the bridge between the activity itself and the community. Without them, there's nothing." We need more!

So David made it easier and quicker for teaching artists to step up. They no longer have to wait for an opening to attend a training in New York City, nor do they have to expense the travel costs. In 2024 David created an on-demand online training curriculum that is coordinated with one-on-one training sessions with a mentor or facilitator. Now people can train on their own schedule from anywhere in the world with limited expense. This has allowed Dance for PD to expand its presence, particularly internationally and in rural areas.

There are two levels of teacher training. The first is the introductory training process where they learn the fundamentals of how to teach the Dance for PD class. Once the teaching artist completes the introductory training either in person or online, they go into community to pilot their teaching.

When teachers are interested and ready, they can return for certification. They must teach at least fifty hours to qualify for certification. That process is designed to measure the quality of their teaching, evaluate their class, and do a peer review of their class by video. Candidates take two online exams, and there is some reflective work. Thirty-eight of the eight hundred active teachers are certified.

"It's like having a master's degree versus a bachelor's degree," explained David. "Certification is the next level. Once they pass all that, they are officially certified and we license their program." At that point they are allowed to use the Dance for PD trademark and brands and are featured on its website. Certification lasts for life, with professional development required every two years. The annual license can be renewed annually if the local program meets the license standards.

If a teacher chooses not to become certified, "It's not like you don't have the skills to teach. A lot of teachers just don't have the time to go through certification, and we don't pressure them. They don't need the brand. They just love what they are doing."

Certified teachers are professional teachers of dance of any style and the license holders are often the institutions that employ them. Current licensees around the world range from sole proprietor studios, dance companies, and presenting organizations like theaters to medical clinics and hospitals. The licensed entity can call their program Dance for PD as long as they have a certified teacher teaching.

Sometimes Dance for PD trains a pool of teachers for a particular area so teachers can rotate, such as in New York City.

In addition, David says there are about 550 trainees from their Educational and Professional Enrichment course who are not in the teacher training track. This course is designed for people without a dance teaching background who want a comprehensive overview of the Dance for PD approach for their own enrichment. Participants might include mental health and physical therapists, caregivers, medical professionals, or people with Parkinson's. Others, including recreational dancers, may wish to assist in classes or become trained assistants in Dance for PD classes. All trainees in the program must have some dance training or dance education.

All good. But having trained teachers and allies is not always enough. There needs to be a bridge between training and program implementation. As Jessica Roeder of Duluth discovered, there's not always an infrastructure like a nonprofit or health organization in a teacher's local community to start a program. It is hard to obtain start-up funding for a program if there is no local track record.

So David and Dance for PD raised funds through individual philanthropy to launch a micro grant program. People who have trained with them can apply for a grant of up to $2,000 to start a pilot program anywhere in the world. That way the teaching artist can establish a track record of community need and obtain testimonials to support applications for further funding. Grants are offered on a revolving basis throughout the year for about ten grant awards per year.

David is also actively working to create more broad access to Dance for PD particularly for underrepresented populations. He is expanding the Dance for PD Spanish language programming and is focusing on building partnerships with the African American community, a community that has traditionally not been drawn to Parkinson's movement activities. To accomplish that, his team is working to ensure the information is available across the clinical landscape, not just with specialists like neurologists, but with general care practitioners, community health care workers, and social workers. The goal is to attract more teaching artists of color and more participants of color in local programming.

Talk about scaling up the community of teaching artists and allies in multiple ways within health care *around the globe*. With start-up funding to boot! It's a brilliant strategy. Replicable, too, for other organizations.

I am personally inspired as a nonprofit founder and leader about the possibilities of engaging with Dance for PD and creating a sustainable structure to support this amazing work in Minnesota. I hope others are inspired to do the same in other states.

Similar possibilities exist for teachers to become trained to bring the benefits of dance to people with dementia, such as through the Dance Vision Foundation, as discussed in Chapter 28. They are currently building their infrastructure to grow their footprint beyond the West Coast and to create their own training opportunity for teachers and dance allies. The success of Dance for PD in creating an educated cadre of teachers and trainers over time may be a model for Dance Vision Foundation and similar organizations around the country.

So here's the bottom line question. Are you a dance professional, amateur dancer, or dance ally who wants to give back in a meaningful way? You can step up now.

And it may become one of the best things you'll ever do in your life.

Chapter 32

⌄

Dance Movement
Meets Psychotherapy

Sometimes the challenges confronting people are not neurological but psychological. Mental health is a growing
concern for all ages. Yes, we know that dance provides physical,
social, and emotional benefits. But in some cases, it can work
wonders as a true mental health therapy.

You can't write stories about the profound mental health and
emotional impact of dance on people's lives without asking
"How?" Especially if you're a dancer and a psychology major,
like me.

My psychology studies never mentioned dance/movement
therapy. But it's real, and it's fascinating. It's the meeting place of
creative movement, body-mind awareness, and psychotherapy.

How can people seemingly heal from health challenges,
overcome trauma or other emotional barriers, make difficult
transitions, or find new purpose in life just by moving their
bodies? What is the science behind these transformations?

Today there are about twelve hundred certified dance/move-
ment therapists (DMTs) in the United States. The field is
dominated by women, with only 4 percent of DMTs being male.

When I set out to find one of these DMTs, the name Michael
Gardos Reid jumped out at me. I knew that name. Not because

he was secretary of the Minnesota chapter of DMTs, but because he's the son of Liz Reid, a woman I loved as a second mother.

Liz was my campaign manager for five elections to the Minnesota Senate. Michael, just a year older than me, probably helped, too, dropping literature for one or two of my campaigns. Last time I saw him was when I eulogized his mother at her celebration of life in December 2017.

I'm convinced Liz had something to do with our reunion.

The Michael Reid I knew long ago had never shown interest in dance. Or so I thought. To my surprise, I learned that Michael started dancing before kindergarten.

The kids in Michael's neighborhood were putting on a skit show. At the time, he was not only the new kid on the block but one of the younger kids as well. He wanted to be part of the show, but there wasn't a part for him. Instead, he was invited to "dance between every skit." So he did.

Later, when the Beatles came to fame during his elementary years, he "went nuts" with his dancing. He described his dance as "ecstatic," not structured.

"During middle school, people told me: 'You shouldn't dance now—that's for later,'" he said. "They were probably jealous because I was having so much fun. Such a wild guy. I just kept dancing and dancing."

Michael attended the University of Minnesota in his twenties but soon dropped out.

"I couldn't figure out which of the ten or twelve things I found most interesting I really want to do," he explained. "I wandered around. Some take a gap year. I took a gap decade. When I left school, I wanted to be a cultural revolutionary, a person who organizes participatory art events, like improv theater or music concerts. But I didn't know how to organize, and I didn't have many mentors. By the end of my twenties, I got physically sick, trying to make things happen without taking care of myself. I was living with lung congestion and probably depression."

Michael tried going back to school a second and even third time, only to drop out again. But the third time, he was motivated to use his fee statement to get books at the university library.

He read psychologist Carl Jung, who talks about the shadow, the part of us we don't want to deal with or relate to. With Jungian theory in his mind, Michael started having intense, violent dreams.

"Finally, I figured out that my dreams symbolized being strongly emotional," Michael said. "I'd been such a nice guy since my high school days, so I needed to develop my ability to disagree with people, to be more firm, angry, and sharp with people. When I came around to that idea, the dreams calmed down, and I popped up like a cork."

He started studying tai chi intensively. He sought counseling, but sitting down in therapy was hard for him.

"I was in my head so much," he said. "I was a very smart kid, so I would overthink everything. I would get more and more depressed when the therapist asked me things. I felt ashamed or stuck. If this had been twenty years later, they probably would have put me on antidepressants."

While studying tai chi, Michael happened upon a woman teaching an introductory dance therapy workshop. He decided he wanted to become a dance therapist. But first, he wanted to get some dance therapy himself. As they say, "Doctor, heal thyself." So he shifted from student to client, attending dance therapy sessions about once a month.

At the first session, the therapist asked, "How are you feeling?"

"I don't know," he replied. "I'm tied up in knots about it."

"So why don't you get up, walk around a little, and see what you find out," she said.

What happened next was a breakthrough on several levels, as Michael recalled: "I got up and took one, two, three steps—and I immediately knew what I was feeling. When you stand up, your breath is more engaged. You're more in action. I process more through my sensations. From the time I was four years old, dance was a primary language for me. If I'm going to express conflicts or difficult emotions, movement is just normal."

The dance therapy sessions were powerful for Michael. "In one session, I knew exactly what I wanted to do," he said. "I wanted to have the therapist sit on one side of the room and not say anything for the first half hour. Not getting verbal was important to me. Then I went to the other side of the room and sat down against the wall. I started moving my hands, almost like painting with my hands on the floor in front of me. It seemed almost like I was pushing out and creating a space around me on the floor. It felt so good. She's watching me. I've got my space, and I'm creating more space for myself. I was the eldest of seven children, and we lived in pretty tight quarters. The idea of having my own space plus this person's singular attention plus the freedom to not have to explain myself somehow added up to what I needed. I could own my space and become my own self."

As the sessions progressed, Michael uncovered an almost universal insight.

"I felt like I wanted to have my therapist's support in a physical way. Though my mother was a very physical person, she tended to be taken up by a new child every couple years. I could often get her ear, but she wasn't able to put her arm around me because she was busy holding a new baby. So I wanted physical support that would be like nurturing me. My therapist and I clarified that we were not trying to be romantic. We worked out where I could lean on her while she sat on the floor, she could give me a hug, or she could let me put my head on her shoulder as a form of expressing 'I've got some support for you.'"

To Michael, this "support" activity highlighted the difference between dance/movement therapy and traditional talk therapy.

"Such a thing would be hard to translate in a verbal psychotherapy session," he said. "If someone just *said* they supported me, I don't know if I would have really believed or absorbed it. But having the physical expression of support in my life, I started to feel able to take risks to have more healthy intimacy in all my relationships. I could start to grow a new romantic relationship, which eventually led to my first wife."

Michael felt empowered. He had a new direction. He was committed to dance/movement therapy. He finished his bachelor's degree at age thirty-two and went on to obtain a master's in arts in counseling psychology and dance/movement therapy from Antioch University New England.

Michael then returned to his Twin Cities roots and was hired as a DMT at Abbott Northwestern Hospital in Minneapolis. Dance/movement therapy had been a core practice in Abbott's mental health unit since 1970. Michael is still there today, over thirty years later. His second wife is an Abbott DMT as well.

At Abbott, Michael provided DMT for people with psychotic disorders in the locked units—people dealing with psychosis, bipolar disorder, severe depression, schizophrenia, suicidality, and aggressive behavior disorders. Then he moved to helping people with anxiety and depression in outpatient mental health programs.

DMT can help two groups of people, as Michael explained. The first group is people uncomfortable expressing themselves verbally or unable to make a verbal representation of their experience. Perhaps they experienced something when they were preverbal or when they lacked verbal understanding. DMT helps this group because it focuses on their nonverbal expression, which may feel more natural for them.

Conversely, the other group is people *too* comfortable expressing themselves verbally. DMT helps these people because it pulls them out of their heads and into their bodies.

"Some of us can give a really good 'show' at therapy," Michael said. "For me, I was overthinking all the time. I was trying to mastermind what my therapy was going to be about."

This is why a dance/movement therapy technique such as Authentic Movement can be so helpful. Developed by DMT Mary Starks Whitehouse, Authentic Movement incorporates movement to promote self-exploration and improved mental health.

"Something like Authentic Movement allows us to go underneath our social shell and get into different parts of ourselves that we might need to visit for various reasons," Michael explained. "But we don't exactly know how to get there on our own because we're so good at looking OK and presenting ourselves to everybody."

In Authentic Movement, one person takes the role of the witness, and the other person takes the role of the mover. The witness offers support by watching the other person's movement process. The mover closes their eyes, listens to their body, and allows movement to unfold spontaneously. The mover doesn't consciously choose to do any particular dance routine, shape, or posture. The mover simply explores emotions and feelings, right then and there. After the time is over, the two reflect on the experience.

Michael has seen the power of Authentic Movement first-hand. "I had a guy come to me who was a former air force pilot, and his father was the same," he began. "The son had this inner war going on: Father wants him to be at least a copilot, if not a pilot, of a commercial airliner, but does the son really want to do that? We did Authentic Movement for a long time, and I supported him and had him listen to himself as he moved: 'If I walk around like a pilot, does that feel like me? Am I faking it? Am I doing it for Dad, more than for me?' He ultimately figured out he was going for copilot. He was finally able to cure and hear himself enough just through moving. He had to get behind the persona of having to present himself in a certain way for the comfort of other people. He was empowered by this. Authentic Movement is an invitation to have a waking dream through movement."

A waking dream through movement. So powerful. Maybe that's why after I eulogized Michael's mother back in 2017, I found myself dancing for her approval for weeks afterwards. She made me smile as I practiced.

Did dancing help me process my grief and my loving memories of Liz? I didn't know anything about dance/movement therapy at the time.

But Michael did. And Liz too.

Chapter 33

Dance Medicine:
Dancing Healthy at All Ages

Hopefully most of us won't experience the specific neuro-logical or psychological challenges we just explored in the previous chapters. But all of us, regardless of age, will experi-ence basic physical challenges, especially if we love to ballroom dance. It's just a matter of time.

It usually goes something like this . . .

You feel pain in your ankle or shoulder or maybe your lower back. It'll go away, right? If you're a professional dancer, you push through because teaching is your livelihood or because your competition career is at risk. If you're a social dancer or amateur competitor, you push through because your passion for dance provides community and purpose in your life. Whoever you are, you keep dancing and ignore the pain.

Until you can't.

Finally, you see your family physician. They advise you to rest and refrain from dancing for weeks or even months. Not what you want to hear. So you keep dancing and ignore their advice *and* the pain.

But once again, the pain gets so bad that you simply can't ignore it. You know you need help. If only you could find a provider who understands you *as a dancer*.

You're in luck.

Dance medicine is a unique specialized field with various medical professionals (physicians, physical therapists, psychologists, and nutritionists, among others) who take care of dancers. Those of us who live in the Twin Cities are extra lucky, as our dance medicine community is a national leader. I discovered that when I sought physical therapy for my own dance ailments in 2022 from Dr. Megin Sabo John, a doctor of physical therapy at Twin Cities Orthopedics.

"I think it's hard with dancers," said Megin. "They're similar to runners. You can't just tell them to stop. If you tell a runner to stop, he'll just go to another person."

A classical ballet performer herself and a lover of African dance and Lindy Hop, Megin knows how to keep people out on the dance floor even as they're recovering and healing.

"As a provider, I can help with a strategy to modify or limit the time dancing," Megin explained. "Maybe dance one hour a day rather than four. Or maybe focus on a particular style of dance because each style has its own demand. It's about negotiating what is healthy participation for the dancer. It's more like running a 5K rather than a marathon."

Megin came to Minnesota about ten years ago to join its thriving dance medicine community. Dr. Brad Moser—a family medicine–trained doctor, classical pianist, and salsa dancer—sparked the dance medicine community in Minnesota around 2004. He was completing a sports medicine fellowship at Hennepin County Medical Center when a professional dancer friend told him, "Brad, if you're in sports medicine, you need to be a go-to dance medicine doctor because there isn't one in town we can trust."

Today, Brad is indeed the go-to dance medicine doctor in the Twin Cities. He's also the founder of the Minnesota Dance Medicine Foundation, where Megin has served on the board of directors. Started in 2009, the foundation serves as a model for dance medicine organizations around the country. (We'll discuss more about the foundation's important mission shortly.)

What makes dance medicine different from other sports medicine?

Brad believes that it's important for dancers to understand that they are athletes. "I call them dancer athletes," Brad said. "You treat them as athletes. You investigate what may occur in that sport versus other sports. There are certain specific things that occur in a dancer that wouldn't occur in a hockey player. For example, a hockey player wears a boot, so the risk of ankle injuries is low. A dancer has a high rate of ankle injuries—from sprains to stress fractures to impingement issues. It's knowing the specificity of the dancer athlete, to know to look for those things when you see them."

Dance medicine providers must approach their dance athlete patients with a different index of suspicion.

"I tell my provider-learners, 'Never let a dancer with back pain leave your office without ruling out a stress fracture,'" Brad said. "It's not stress or sprain—they wouldn't be in there for that. Dancers are some of the toughest athletes I've ever taken care of. They are very dedicated to their sport, and they just push through. So if a dancer has had back pain for a while, you need further imaging to sort out whether there is a stress fracture."

Dance medicine providers earn patients' trust because they understand the language of dance.

"With my background, dance is the language I speak," Megin said. "I relate to dancers because I understand what their training schedule is like. When you talk about ballet in particular, there's a lot of vocabulary that goes with it. I get a lot of buy-in from the patient. They believe I understand their sport or passion or career. It's very rewarding. They're thankful for your services and that you understand what they do for a living. It's different than going to a sports medicine provider who specializes in football—they might not understand the specific demand on the dancer body."

Dance medicine providers especially know how to use a dancer's age as a critical guide for care. For example, they advise that youth and adolescents should not dance more than their age in hours per week.

"If you're sixteen and dancing twenty-five hours per week, you're dancing too many hours for what your body can handle," Megin explained. "We have to educate young dancers and get buy-in from them and their parents. Their frontal lobe is not fully developed yet, and their decision-making abilities are not there."

"We know from research that if a young athlete is exercising greater than his age in hours per week, the injury rate goes up exponentially," Brad added. "That's well proven. They have to be aware that there will be a significantly increased injury rate in those dancers."

As adolescents transition into adulthood, however, dance medicine providers can help them safely scale up their efforts. That's because once the human skeleton matures, growth plates close and bones fully develop.

"Then we're looking at 'loading' over time," Megin said. "If you start dancing at ten hours per week, and you want your end range at forty hours per week, you have to build up slowly to that. You can't jump from ten to forty hours in a week, or you'll have an overuse injury."

For adult dancers, one of the biggest concerns is to listen to their bodies and get things checked out early if there's a problem.

"That way, people like Megin and myself can make sure we're nipping that minor injury very fast, so it doesn't become a bigger injury," Brad said.

Dance medicine providers also understand that new concerns arise once a dancer moves into middle age.

"We have a very active population in the Twin Cities," Brad said. "So we have active middle-aged people come in and say, 'Hey, doc—why does my Achilles hurt so bad?' 'Well, how old are you, Jim?' 'About fifty.' 'Well, so is your Achilles tendon!' We help the patient understand they won't heal as well as a fifteen-year-old. The integrity and healing potential of the tendon is just not as good as it was back then. They may be overusing it."

Megin often supports aging dance athletes with physical therapy exercises to prevent injury and to prevent or relieve pain. Frequent dancing, particularly if the dancer repeats movements over and over, puts great demand on the body. Sometimes forty-year-old dance teachers have the type of hip arthritis that is usually found in senior citizens.

"The reality is, your body is slowly deteriorating as you age, and you have to support it," Megin said. "You want to add balance exercises and strength training. You have to work your cardio. You have to work on your recovery tools, whether that's massage, Epsom salt baths, massage guns, or foam rollers. You must do all the support work to make your body healthy enough that you can keep doing it day after day." Megin also advises that if a woman is losing bone density, she needs to support her bone health to prevent osteoporosis.

What is the most vulnerable body area for the middle-aged ballroom dancer? According to Megin, it's the upper thoracic spine.

"How much extension do you have there?" she asked. "If you want a bigger look, you will get it from somewhere else, which may engage the lower back. You need core strength to support that leaning position, so you're not just holding onto your partner but you're meeting your partner where he is. You're supporting your own body."

Shoulders are also vulnerable in adult ballroom dancers.

"If you're not working to prevent impingement, with good shoulder and upper back exercises, you may end up with significant pain," Brad explained. "This is no different than if someone decides to paint his entire house who has never done it before. If you paint over and over, that will impinge the shoulder. If you're untrained or aren't doing enough ballroom dance and come in cold, you're probably going to have an impingement shoulder issue."

Finally, what about the senior citizen dancer? An elder dancer may have a seventy-year-old rotator cuff with a partial tear. Or they may have arthritis in the shoulder or neck that started long ago and progressed over time.

"I think the older dancer needs to understand that if she has pain, it's not just because she's dancing more," Brad explained. "She needs to get specificity of the diagnosis so we can treat it better. That may mean, for example, an injection in the arthritic shoulder joint."

Older dancers should also be careful when learning new skills.

"Your body will respond to a new movement with pain, dysfunction, or limitations," Megin said. "You wake up sore—is it good sore or bad sore? Can you work through it? It's important to understand good pain versus bad pain, chronic pain versus acute pain."

So, what are a few specific dance medicine strategies for older dancers? To start, don't skip the warm-up.

"If you go cross-country skiing in Minnesota, nobody warms up—but they should," Megin said. "Dancers do the same thing. But dance itself shouldn't be the warm-up. And you can't just dance. You have to do some supplemental things, whether strength training, sleeping, nutrition, and all of the recovery work. There's a lot of independent time that comes in managing your body. I try to teach my patients how to do that. That's the ownership of being able to then do the work."

Translation: If we choose to dance, it's up to us to remain healthy as individuals and partners in dance. That's a personal call to action for each of us dancers, whether we're younger or older, beginner or veteran.

Megin tells her clients, "You must advocate for yourself. You're the only one who knows how you feel."

A large component of dance medicine focuses on helping dancers of all ages make educated decisions based on expert resources, specialists, and experience with outcomes. This is especially true for professional or upcoming dancers. When these dancers are sidelined with injuries, they're probably not getting paid, and they're definitely not progressing toward their goals. But dance medicine providers can help broaden their options.

Brad shared examples from his practice. An exceptional Twin Cities high school ballet dancer received a scholarship to a prestigious New York City ballet school. However, he was experiencing serious pain with his ankles, restricting his range of motion. X-rays revealed two large bones in the back of his ankles.

Brad determined that unless the bones were removed, the young dancer would continue to have pain and restriction. But removing the bones would force the dancer to take time off for recovery, and it could jeopardize his scholarship—and his future dreams. It was a difficult decision.

Brad helped him decide to remove the bones, despite the recovery downtime. The dancer asked the school to defer his admission for a year, with the doctor's assurance that he would come back pain-free and better. The school agreed. Today, the young man is still a professional dancer in New York City.

A similar story occurred with a New York City ballerina who was originally from the Twin Cities. A bone needed to be removed in her big toe. With advice from Brad and colleagues, the ballerina informed the NYC ballet that she would have surgery but come back better than ever after recovery. After six months of rehabilitation, she returned pain-free and worked back to her previous level of dance.

"This is another example," Brad said, "of understanding where the dancer is going, where they are in their career, and making sure they're getting to where they want to go through specific procedures or little surgeries."

In short, it's another example of the power of dance medicine.

"You need to help us help you," Brad said. "If you trust us, we'll get you there."

Prevention of physical injury and wise decision-making are essential parts of dance medicine. But dance medicine focuses on many more components and strategies that enable dancers of all genres, ages, and abilities to be healthy. In fact, "Dance Healthy" is the mission of the nonprofit Minnesota Dance Medicine Foundation (MDMF).

"Dance Healthy" means more than most dancers may realize. Maybe you warm up a few minutes before you step on the dance floor. Maybe you take a few days off when you pull your hamstring, or you change your dance shoes to relieve foot pain. All good. But are you eating the right foods and hydrating? Are you working on strength training off the dance floor, especially as you age? Are you calming the anxieties arising from competitions or comparison with other dancers? Are you *really* dancing healthy?

To Brad, "Dance Healthy" has great meaning. "It's about listening to your body and understanding the resources available to you when you think something isn't feeling right," he explained. "It's a way to inform dancer athletes of any age that it's important to understand their bodies, understand that injuries can happen and are preventable, that nutrition is imperative and hydration important. Whether it's the medical side with physicians, physical therapists, or trainers or the nutrition side or the mental health side with suicide prevention and eating disorders, the links on the website are an important community resource."

MDMF uses collegial educational conferences to teach dancers about their health as well as to educate medical providers about dance medicine. Sometimes the MDMF taps national experts to provide insight. MDMF also operates a free clinic for dancers in downtown Minneapolis, where dancers, who are often underinsured, receive treatment from volunteer professional health care providers.

There are numerous online resources written by dance medicine providers at www.mndancemed.org. These resources can help dancers of all ages and genres. Topics include rehabilitation following injury, mental health supports, nutrition for injury prevention and healing, and treating acute injuries.

While MDMF has focused most of its efforts in Minnesota, the foundational principles and online resources apply anywhere. Dance medicine entities of various types exist in other areas of the country such as Seattle, Atlanta, and Denver, to name a few. Might more health providers in other states adopt this vision?

Coincidentally, the dance medicine vision is currently alive and well on the island of Maui in Hawaii. In 2023, after twelve years in Minnesota working with performing artists, Megin chose a lifestyle change and moved to Maui with her husband because they wanted scuba diving to be a greater part of their life together. Megin "handed the reins" of her Twin Cities clinical practice in dance medicine to others, including her membership on the Minnesota Dance Medicine Foundation board.

But the dancers of Maui are the winners here. Today Megin is working with local adolescent studio dancers and adult dancers in her new clinic position at Imua Physical Therapy. "The dance community has been welcoming and appreciative to have a specialist on the island," said Megin.

So here's an opportunity for health providers around the nation: Why not create a similar dance medicine foundation or service organization to support the dance community in your state or region?

And for all dancers of any style, experience, or age, here's your personal call to action: If you choose to take care of yourself and dance healthy, you truly can dance until the end with purpose and joy.

All good. But so much more can be done. How can *you* join the Dance of Resilience?

A far more comprehensive Call to Action awaits in Part VI.

PART VI

Call to Action

This is an urgent call to action.

- **We need government and philanthropic funders** to step up support for critical research with innovative technologies that measure the impact of dance and art activities on the human brain.
- **We need insurance companies and medical institutions** to promote the benefits of neuroarts and invest directly in dance and arts opportunities for members and patients.
- **We need community leaders (federal, state, and local policymakers; health entities and agencies; and foundations and nonprofits)** to invest in community-based whole person health and well-being, including social prescribing and Community as Medicine models to ensure that the benefits of dance and the arts are available equitably to all, regardless of resources.

Why do we need this action?

So thousands more people may live healthier lives, and so we can lower health care costs for all.

It's already in motion. All we need is you.

Chapter 34

Call to Action for Research and Support for Neuroarts

Virtually every story in this book demonstrates how music and dance can improve our physical, mental, and emotional health and help us prevent, manage, or overcome disease challenges. While these stories serve as anecdotal evidence, they align with the vast body of science-based knowledge and evidence accumulating over many disciplines about the benefits of dance.

"What we're seeing, I think, is a deeper acceptance of the benefits of dance within the Parkinson's community and the medical community," said David Leventhal, cofounder of Dance for PD. "There's still a bit of a climb, but I think we've gotten over the big hump of people not understanding or accepting what dance can do. They see the research. They hear it from the medical community. They see it broadly in programs like Sound Health, a collaboration between the National Institutes of Health and the Kennedy Center, and in the NeuroArts Blueprint." (We'll discuss this more below.) "Doctors are acknowledging that we need complementary programming like Dance for PD to provide the kind of biopsychosocial support that medicine and surgery alone can't.

And I think that even in the last two years, that realization has become more profound."

This is great news, but there's much more to be done. While working on this book, I interviewed several accomplished leaders in arts and sciences around the country, only to discover that these leaders often weren't aware that others were doing similar work in their field. In some cases, I introduced them to one another.

Yes, the work connecting brain science and arts has been impressive and robust. But it's also been fragmented.

Thankfully, some are setting out to change that.

Created in 2019, the NeuroArts Blueprint: Advancing the Science of Arts, Health and Wellbeing initiative (www.neuro-artsblueprint.org) is a partnership between the International Arts + Mind Lab at Johns Hopkins University School of Medicine's Center for Applied Neuroaesthetics and the Aspen Institute's Health, Medicine and Society Program. The initiative's goal is to create a collective power through the arts to improve the health and well-being of individuals and communities.

In December 2021, the initiative launched the Blueprint, a network of researchers, art practitioners, artists, community leaders, and other allies who understand the imperative of using art as a science-based tool to advance our collective health and well-being. It's a "neuroarts ecosystem," where research can be stored and translated into practice for clinics, homes, work-places, and communities. Implementation is underway to scale up research, training, and practice components within the field.[1]

The Blueprint outlines its own call to action to build a fully recognized field of research and practice, scale up and sustain programming and practices with dedicated funding, enact sup-portive public and private sector policies, and educate and train the workforce and leaders within the ecosystem. It's no surprise that David Leventhal is a member of the Advisory Council.

Smaller breakthrough strategies that integrate the benefits of dance and arts programming into health and well-being are already underway in the public and private domains. But to grow this ecosystem on a larger scale, we need two things: 1) specific research and data around brain science and dance that will incentivize the health care community and 2) community engagement.

We'll discuss community engagement in the final two chapters. But first, let's talk research.

New Fields of Research

As David explains, multiple research studies have connected neuroscience and dance over the years, but they've only been preliminary or smaller-scale projects.

"They're important as a ramp-up to the larger-scale studies," he said. "But we haven't seen the large-cohort studies that we'd like to see. Those are expensive."

In the next five years, David hopes to see a multicenter study around the impact of dance on Parkinson's, particularly as it relates to motor skill, quality of life, and reduction of fall risk.

"Falls are so detrimental to quality of life and morbidity and mortality numbers," he added. "They're the most acute cause of hospitalization among people with Parkinson's. If we could reduce those numbers considerably, we'd improve quality of life for people with PD and reduce the burden on health care providers."

That is, if studies could show that dance reduces fall risk for people with PD (a result that other studies have shown for other populations), then perhaps more health care providers, insurance companies, and federal, state, and local health agencies would honor dance as an effective low-cost care option for people with PD. Fewer falls would significantly reduce the burden on the health care system.

This is a more traditional research approach, to zero in on an easily measurable physical effect of a specific disorder. But new research modalities have emerged in recent years that can contribute important information into health challenges well beyond Parkinson's. David is especially encouraged by what he's seeing from the new generation of neurologists.

"They've been trained in the context of a more holistic model for Parkinson's," he said.

David and his teams at Dance for PD and Mark Morris Dance Center are working with two researchers in particular, with funding mechanisms designed to eventually ramp up.

The first researcher is Dr. Aston McCullough, MPhil, PhD, assistant professor with Northeastern University's Department of Physical Therapy, Movement, and Rehabilitation Science and a core faculty member of their Center for Cognitive and Brain Health.

"We're working on a project funded through the National Institutes of Health that looks at the impact of dance on physical activity measures," David said. "We know that dance positively impacts a number of outcomes, but little is known about the physical activity intensities that led to those outcomes. By looking at outputs like oxygen uptake and heart rate in those participating in both group classes and at home via Zoom, we can start to develop an algorithm to train physical activity classifiers to detect the absolute and relative physical activity intensities of Dance for PD sessions. That can then inform how we might design Dance for PD interventions so that benefits are more consistent and replicable across the population."

David hopes they can build on the study in collaboration with Dr. McCullough and apply for more funding for a larger multicenter study in the future.

The second researcher David's team is working with is Dr. Constantina Theofanopoulou, a dancer, neuroscientist, and research assistant professor at Rockefeller University. She's using magnetic resonance imaging (MRI) to observe the changes that occur in our brains when we dance.

"In some ways, this is the gold standard," David explained, "because it helps us to understand the mechanisms of change. We know that dance is effective by looking at external outcomes such as walking speed, balance, depression, social isolation, and other measures. But what we don't understand is *why* dance does this. If you can see what's happening in the brain as a result of dance activity, then we can say these things are happening because the brain is rewiring itself or because certain parts of the brain are being activated as a result of dance activity—and not because of other activity."

Dr. Theofanopoulou is currently part of a research team using brain caps to capture the brain activity of five dancers as they engage in a sixty-minute performance of butoh. Butoh is a form of Japanese dance theater that involves extremely slow movements. MRI generally requires patients to keep their heads motionless, so butoh makes this research possible in a way other dance forms wouldn't.

This is a highly complex form of research. Dance involves many interrelated regions in the brain—sensory, motor, cognitive, social, emotional, rhythmic, and creative—that all need to be observed. That may be why most current Parkinson's research is focused on only the biochemistry of Parkinson's and is conducted through a pharmacological or surgical lens.

Not to mention, MRI research is very expensive. One MRI could cost at least $1,500. A major funding source is needed to scale this up. But the potential benefits from this research are far greater than the costs. This research could build a platform for understanding how the brain really works for dance and beyond.

Dr. Theofanopoulou's interest in the neurobiology of dance arises from her graduate work studying the neural pathways of singing behavior in birds. She identified an intriguing correlation as relayed on her website: "Humans and parrots, the only species capable of synchronized body movements to a beat, an important component of what we call 'dance,' are also the ones that possess the most advanced vocal learning abilities in the animal kingdom."[2]

David sees the potential this way: "If we can understand how birds create very complex patterns using their voices, that gives us an understanding of how the brain controls those sounds. We share a common ancestor with birds, hundreds of millions of years ago. We're one of the only other animals that can consciously create a very broad range of song. So what's the relationship between a bird's brain and a human brain? How can we apply that to dance and movement? Parrots can respond to a rhythmic beat as humans can. Have you ever seen a cockatoo rocking to the beat? So how do we build those scientific correlations? And how can we use that to understand a healthy human brain and a brain that is living with a condition like Parkinson's?"

Good questions. We need this research to continue.

Here's our Call to Action:

- We need major state and federal health agencies and private foundations to step up and fund important research in the neuroarts venue that focuses on the neural mechanics of change, not just the existence of change.
- We need investment from private sources and public entities such as the National Science Foundation and the National Institutes of Health to sponsor multicenter, large-cohort mechanistic studies to build the body of unrefuted scientific evidence that illustrate the benefits of dance on brain health.

"That will allow us to achieve what large institutions and the medical profession are asking for," said David. "We have all the preliminary research out there. I think we need to step up to the next level. This kind of support allows us to move the needle on a larger scale."

And once that support happens, an entire community will be awaiting, ready to engage.

Chapter 35

⌄

Call to Action for Social Prescribing: From Policymakers to Health Insurers

Now section chief of the Cleveland Clinic's Center for Geriatric Medicine, Dr. Ardeshir Hashmi once had a ninety-three-year-old patient who complained of excruciating chest pains. The odd thing was, her symptoms always seemed to disappear once she was around medical staff, even as she received extensive medical workups.

After two years and nearly fifty emergency room visits, the lightbulb went off for Dr. Hashmi. He realized that the woman was simply feeling anxious. She lived alone and had no support or reassurance for her anxiety.

Feeling like he was out of medical options, he referred the woman to a geriatric social worker, who helped her enroll in ballroom dance classes.

"Incredibly, the dancing started and the emergency visits stopped," he said.

Her social worker drove her to dance lessons, swayed with her in her chair to jazzy swing, and reconnected her with her love of music and her friends at the community center.[1]

Pills were not the answer for this patient. In effect, the doctor had written her a social prescription for ballroom dance classes.

There are many models of social prescribing. Generally, a social prescription targets social health, which a growing number of health providers believe is as important to address as physical or mental health. The value of this approach is gaining momentum at a time when the US Surgeon General and others have observed an epidemic of loneliness.

A formal social prescribing model typically connects patients with community-focused activities customized to their interests, such as group exercise, dance, art classes, outdoor activities, and volunteer opportunities.

"That means really digging in to understand each patient's interests and personal priorities—the things they live for," Dr. Hashmi explained in a *Cleveland Clinic Consult QD* article.[2]

Think of the possibilities here to integrate partner dance, the arts, and all things community into the health care system!

Over twenty other countries have adopted social prescribing, with England being the earliest. Indeed, the National Health Service in England is the only major health care system that has funded social prescribing nationally. And both the United Kingdom and Japan even have loneliness ministers that administer social prescribing programs.

A key component of the British system is the link worker, a nonmedical professional who can collaborate with a physician to facilitate the patient's participation in a particular activity. The link worker may help find ways to cover costs, register the patient for classes, or arrange transportation. They're also the accountability component of the system, as they follow up to assure the patient's participation and to coordinate with the doctor to monitor outcomes.

Most other countries have developed their systems of social prescribing within the realm of socialized medicine. Unfortunately, the United States is lagging behind in social prescribing. Why?

"Ours is the most complicated system," explained Dr. Alan Siegel, executive director and cofounder of Social Prescribing

USA (www.socialprescribingusa.com). "We have nine hundred health care systems, not just one main system, with other smaller insurers for wealthy people. Most of our system is not government run. Only about 30 percent of it is run by Medicaid and Medicare. The rest of it is private insurers."

But this hasn't stopped Alan from trying to build a social prescribing system in the United States. It's no wonder that Alan also has been a self-described social prescriber for over twenty years. A California family physician, Alan has been a musician since middle school and has played guitar in various bands for years.

He's led various performance events at hospitals, including some called Healing through Creativity, where staff members express their artistic talents. He's also created arts and health programs of multiple modalities in the context of private health hospitals and networks. These initiatives have included Saturday workshops for stress reduction, a farmers market in the hospital, and an expressive arts therapy program that could be delivered bedside, at a hospital, in group medical visits, in community, and even at homeless shelters.

Since COVID, Alan has been motivated to help health care workers suffering from burnout. He wants to bring arts to these practitioners to lessen their stress and help them deal with the reality that there will be fewer health care workers in the future.

"We're at the point that we need to do something different from multiple angles," Alan said. "We have a health worker crisis. Twenty-five percent of people have already left health care. They're expecting another 20 percent to leave in the next two years. We'll be in trouble when it comes. We won't have enough people to provide health care."

According to Alan, that reality creates pressure to make things happen, especially because the health care crisis coincides with the civic crisis of people not being engaged in community.

"Community involvement has decreased at least 75 percent in the last twenty or thirty years," he said.

In 2022, Alan heard a podcast by Jill Sonke, research director at the University of Florida's Center for Arts in Medicine. (More on her below.) It inspired him to collaborate with social entrepreneur Dan Morse to cocreate Social Prescribing USA. The nonprofit serves as a national voice to bring visibility for the field, connect local organizations engaged in this work, identify best practices, prioritize policy development and advocacy, and build a national group of implementers, including physicians, to put social prescribing into practice.

Today there are more than forty social prescription pilot programs providing services around the country. Some of these pilots serve large constituencies, which creates a solid foundation to sell the strategy of social prescribing more widely, particularly to state, federal, and private health partners.

Here are just three initiatives that launched in 2024.

One initiative saw Massachusetts launch the first statewide social prescribing solution in the United States. It's a partnership between Art Pharmacy, the Mass Cultural Council, and Mass General Brigham.

According to a June 27, 2024, press release, Georgia-based Art Pharmacy's services enabled health care providers and other care team members to prescribe arts and culture participation to individuals with a range of health concerns. Following a three-year pilot, the Mass Cultural Council selected Art Pharmacy to build a network of arts and culture organizations, recruit additional institutional stakeholders, and build sustainable relationships with health systems and health plans in Massachusetts. More than three hundred cultural organizations signed with Art Pharmacy for this work.

In the press release, Michael J. Bobbitt, executive director of the Mass Cultural Council, stated, "We know this work to be effective preventive medicine and are thrilled it will also create a new revenue stream for cultural organizations who—for the first time—will be compensated specifically for the health benefits they provide. This is a creative way to advance the creative and cultural sector in Massachusetts and leverage the benefits of arts participation for the greater good."[3]

In another initiative, Stanford University—in partnership

with Art Pharmacy—launched the first comprehensive social prescription program available for students by any major university or educational institution.

Commencing January 1, 2024, and working with Vaden Health Services, the goal of this initiative is to address student well-being and reduce crisis care. Vaden's well-being coaches or student-life staff members refer students to Art Pharmacy's care navigators. Care navigators help identify the students' wellness goals and arts interests, and then they match the students with monthly arts and culture experiences on campus, called "doses."

All students are eligible without referral from a physician. Stanford covers all activity-related expenses, including tickets, transportation, and additional accommodations. Each prescription is good for the rest of the academic year at no cost to participants.

In a *Stanford Report* article, Chris Appleton, founder and chief executive officer of Art Pharmacy, detailed the need for the program: "Anxiety, depression, and suicidal ideation rates on college campuses are at an all-time high while mental health providers nationwide are overwhelmed. Introducing non-stigmatized, readily available mental health interventions is critical to reducing suffering amongst college students."[4]

Yet another initiative is a partnership between the New Jersey Performing Arts Center (NJPAC), Horizon Blue Cross and Blue Shield of New Jersey, and the Newark Department of Health and Community Wellness. It's the first social prescribing program in the country to have an insurance carrier as a key partner.

This initiative received an unprecedented grant of $150,000 from the National Endowment for the Arts. The partnership, called ARTS Rx, offers free referrals to arts programs for those coping with anxiety, depression, loneliness, and caregiving stress. Newark residents as well as students at Rutgers University–Newark are eligible to participate.[5]

While these three initiatives focus on multiple arts modalities, I can't help but think of what they could offer people who want a social prescription to partner dance—especially people who do not have resources to afford it. Ballroom dance could become a reality for many participants—from geriatric elders to freshman college students.

The possibilities are exciting. Dance as a social prescription can not only offer better health and physical well-being for individuals but also lower health care costs over time for all of us.

But here's the catch. As of 2025, only about forty US social prescribing sites existed in partnership with individual institutions or government payors. Each pilot was created individually, with much effort to develop a local infrastructure. It's almost like reinventing the wheel with each payor and each medical institution.

How can we expand and scale up in a more efficient way? How can we grow beyond individual pilot programs and create a national social prescribing system in the United States?

"That is the million-dollar question," Alan said.

He's personally walking the walk by working to build a social prescribing system within California-based Kaiser Permanente, where he practices. Kaiser Permanente is an extensive medical network that includes a nonprofit health plan of over twelve million members, forty hospitals, and six hundred medical offices in multiple states.

"But my plan is to make this available for everybody," he said. "I think it'll make the leap when we have real data."

Some real data will arrive soon. Remember Dr. Jill Sonke, the director of research initiatives at the University of Florida Center for Arts in Medicine? She's currently overseeing a major research evaluation project of twenty-three social prescription programs of differing models across the country. Evaluation results are expected in 2025.

That will help. But the most critical data needed for social prescription programs to make that giant leap across the country is solid economic data.

"We need economic data to show the return on investment," Alan said. "We have to prove to a health care insurer that this is an investment worth making. We have to be seen as problem solvers who can save money in the system. We need outcomes built into a system, not just the outcomes of someone going to a dance class. What does this mean for me as a practitioner to refer somebody? How does this really work when you build it into a health care system? We need deeper experience to be able to sell it more widely."

That may take time, especially because we need research and data based in the United States. Data from abroad doesn't apply here, as our health care system is different from that of other countries.

It'll also take money—money that hasn't yet been available. Nearly everything Social Prescribing USA has done so far has been done on a volunteer basis. With proper funding, they could really mobilize their team and push toward their bigger goals.

"We need full-time staff members to support this effort," Alan said. "Every time we conduct a webinar or interact with the public, there's so much enthusiasm and excitement. People come to us all the time asking 'What can we do?' We want to use this energy to make change. We need to professionalize what we're doing as a national organization through individual philanthropy or through strategic partnerships."

Currently, much of the work supporting social prescribing in the United States is based on philanthropy. That's often how system transformation starts. But I see a ray of hope on the horizon.

Recently, the Federal Reserve Bank of New York prioritized social prescribing as a key area of community involvement over a several-year period. Social Prescribing USA participated in a summit with the Federal Reserve leaders and important stake-holders to explore how to sustain this work with major financial investment so they can spread the initiative across the country.

This is a promising partnership. You can't underestimate the influence and fundraising connections that can result from collaboration with the Federal Reserve. I saw this firsthand during the 1990s, when I was a Minnesota state senator. The Federal Reserve Bank of Minneapolis conducted groundbreaking research that showed the significant long-term economic benefits of investing in early-childhood initiatives. The person who led that research—and dramatically changed the conversation about the importance of investing in our youngest children—was none other than Dr. Art Rolnick, the dancer you met in Chapter 20. A helpful coincidence?

Yes, as Alan says, we need to do something different. Here is the Call to Action:

- We need more policymakers to invest in state and local health and arts agencies, such as the Mass Cultural Council and the Newark Department of Health and Community Wellness, to deliver the proven health benefits of social prescribing in community.
- We need more health insurance plans, such as Horizon Blue Cross and Blue Shield of New Jersey, to fund these cost-effective social prescriptions, particularly on a regional or national level.
- We need more hospitals and medical clinics, such as Mass Brigham General and Kaiser Permanente, to step up as role models to help make social prescribing a reality for all.
- We need more higher-education institutions, such as Stanford and Rutgers–Newark, to make this important social prescription investment in their students.
- We need more organizations such as Art Pharmacy to connect the health system to local arts communities to facilitate social prescription.

Finally, we need more community health and well-being models like Community as Medicine. That's the health coaching model Open Source Wellness has created and implemented in California and beyond. Their model is helping lead the way in delivering health and wellness in community.

And don't we all need community?

That's next.

Chapter 36

‿

Call to Action for Community Health and Well-Being

Yes, I'm a dancer, but I'm also a former eighteen-year state senator. Many laws my colleagues and I passed in Minnesota helped groups of individuals. But the most impactful changes we made as legislators happened when we created new opportunities for whole communities or even the people of our entire state.

So consider this chapter a platform for advocacy and change. Not just because I want every one of you to experience the proven benefits of partner dance that the storytellers in this book have shared. No. It's also because I want our health system to recognize that activities like partner dance are essential to whole-person health and well-being.

That's just one small example of community-based wellness. If we're going to address the whole person—each person's physical, mental, emotional, and social needs—then we need to make community-based whole-person wellness an anchor of our health care system.

As discussed in the previous chapter, social prescription is one proven way to bring the community into health care. There are other community-based models as well.

We start here with Community as Medicine, which has nearly a decade of results behind it. This model is helping show the way for other partners and stakeholders to engage the community in whole-person health and well-being.

We have a long way to go to transform our pill-based US health care system. But effective community models and partnerships are emerging and showing results. Your advocacy will help make them part of the mainstream.

I concede that much of this chapter isn't about dance at all. It goes well beyond dance. But it describes a mission that dancers can certainly get behind. It describes a larger movement that those who want to dance can enthusiastically support. It sets forth a mission that *anyone* can get behind who wants a health care system to better meet all our basic human needs.

Join me in dreaming big.

Community as Medicine: A Leading Community Wellness Model

What if you could write your *own* prescription and have a community around you to help you complete it? Maybe a prescription to walk around the block five times every day. A prescription to try a new vegetable. Or a prescription to try a dance class or a movement class at your local YMCA.

It's happening. And it's just getting started.

Dr. Elizabeth (Liz) Markle, a psychologist and professor of community health, was working in clinical health care in California when she became present to a major gap in the health care system.

"As health providers, we all had the best of intentions, telling people to exercise more, to eat better, or to reduce their stress," Liz said. "We gave them 'behavioral prescriptions,' then told them 'Good luck with that. I'll see you in six months.' We were sending people out with prescriptions to nowhere—behavioral prescriptions that no pharmacy in the world can fill."

Liz believed it was no longer ethical to participate in a system where physicians gave behavioral prescriptions that relied on patient privilege and resources to make good on them. So in 2016, she teamed up with Dr. Benjamin Emmert-Aronson in cofounding Open Source Wellness (OSW) (www.opensource-wellness.org) to create an accessible "delivery system" for those prescriptions.

That same year, they created their first Community as Medicine groups in federally qualified health centers in Alameda County, California. Their vision was to create opportunity for doctors, therapists, and other providers to say something like this: "I'm going to write you a prescription. But it's not for medication. It's for participation in a community."

That's a profound idea, especially when research shows that loneliness and lack of social connection are reaching "epidemic" levels in our country. It's also profound that it focuses on community *and* whole-person health and wellness.

"We have four pillars," Liz began. "We say, 'Move, Nourish, Connect, and Be.'"

The Community as Medicine model is a specific form of social prescribing, though with a unique approach. It might be helpful to differentiate it here.

As discussed in the previous chapter, the original social prescribing model is generally built around a link worker, an intermediary who helps the individual navigate between care providers and local arts resources. But resources may be limited in some communities. And some people may not have the ability to visit or feel comfortable in an art museum, dance class, or national park, so they need something that is less of a leap.

Community as Medicine is different. It relies on coaches facilitating group meetings instead of relying on link workers connecting to arts resources.

"The health and wellness coaches are the heart of this," Liz explained. "They have both health and wellness knowledge and deep skills in facilitating interpersonal dynamics. That's the magic of this model. It's not what an expert tells the group participants from the front of the room. It's how they're connected with their peers, who may or may not share the same diagnosis or demographics. They're guided to create a culture of vitality, joy, vulnerability, humanity, and being together with our strengths and challenges."

The coaching approach produced a financial challenge, however. Currently, coaches are not directly reimbursable under Medicaid or Medicare. But Liz and Ben devised a solution.

"In 2017, we learned how to deliver this model as a group medical visit," Liz said. "That was a key turning point for financial sustainability. Coaches are not directly reimbursable, but if you bring in a primary care provider who does short individual medical visits throughout the group, then you have a revenue-generating proposition. What we do is essentially double the billing productivity of that primary care provider because they're not doing the relationship building, the motivational interviewing, or the delivery of information. They're just doing what only they can do."

This funding model works in federally qualified health centers. But other funding strategies must be pursued for other models. In some places, there's community health worker billing. In other places, there's state and private health care transformation dollars that allow tapping into insurer funding. In still other places, there's philanthropy, which may be focused on chronic disease, mental health, and/or social isolation. As the strategies shift, the field shifts. Currently, partnerships are helping to build impact and transform the field. (More on that shortly.)

So, what happens at a Community as Medicine meeting?

Each group consists of between twelve and twenty-five participants and two to four coaches. The participants come together, quickly review group agreements, and do icebreakers. Then they do physical movement for fifteen to twenty minutes.

And yes, the movement is dance based. It's playful.

"It's less about getting a workout and more about laughing and connecting and mirroring each other and being in joy," Liz continued. "Then the group sits down, and there's some sort of stress-reduction practice. Then there's what we call a 'spark,' an interactive educational topic of the day. It might be about cooking well, eating healthy on a budget, setting boundaries in interpersonal relationships, or how to engage in physical movement with your kids."

At this point, the large group splits into small groups of one coach to five or six participants.

"There's about thirty minutes of small-group-coaching time," Liz said. "Individuals are guided to speak about what's going on in their world. They might talk about health, their families, their trauma. At the end of the small-group time, every participant writes a prescription for themselves. The coaches ask, 'What would make a difference for you?' 'What matters to you?' It's that old shift from 'What's the matter *with* you?' to 'What matters *to* you?' We provide little prescription pads, where every participant writes what they are committing to for their well-being for the coming week."

The group closes with affirmations and declarations. It reconvenes in a week. Participants stay connected during the week through a text thread, so there's continuous support and accountability.

"That's what a Community as Medicine group looks like," Liz said. "A starting prescription is twelve weeks of it. In the future I hope it is covered not only by Medicaid and Medicare but the national commercial insurers as well—just like they cover antibiotics or psychotherapy."

Liz describes Community as Medicine as proximal to a clinic. Most people come to the group because they have a prescription from their provider. In fact, a group might meet right in a clinic—or in a doctor's office, in a community setting, or virtually. The meeting may be conducted in English, Spanish, or another language, based on the community. It's all designed to make it as easy as possible for people to participate.

For years, OSW has been gathering data on Community as Medicine's impact. From the start, they knew they had to build an evidence base, so Ben, as a statistician, began to evaluate this work. Liz shared some of this in her November 17, 2023, TEDx talk.

"Our participants see significant increases in physical activity and fruit and vegetable intake. They see massive drops in blood pressure, depression, anxiety, and social isolation. And the figure that really gets the attention of our health insurance partners is that we're seeing about a 77 percent reduction in emergency department visits."[1]

The audience erupted in spontaneous applause. You can't beat that kind of outcome.

Check out the specific data on their website: Participants showed a 51 percent increase in physical activity, a 43 percent decrease in depression, a 19 percent decrease in blood pressure, and a 20 percent reduction in social isolation. No wonder the emergency room visits are decreasing![2]

So far, over five thousand people have participated in Community as Medicine groups with OSW. That's a good start. But only a start.

As Liz said in her TEDx talk, "I dream of the day when it's just as easy to walk into your local Community as Medicine group as it is to walk into a CVS. I dream of the day that you could take your entire family, maybe two nights a week . . . to your local YMCA or community center or church or temple or mosque, wherever it is that you already feel comfortable, and get these four things woven into your evening joyfully, easily. Not because you're showing up with a lot of cash or because you're exerting a ton of willpower, but because we as a society have chosen to invest in and design [opportunities] for these four things that human beings appear to be hardwired to need to be well."[3]

The audience members enthusiastically agreed.

Scaling Up Community as Medicine through Partnerships

When I discovered Open Source Wellness, I imagined great potential to scale up their Community as Medicine model to engage people across the country. But I also knew how difficult it is to scale up anything new in a large system such as US health care.

Despite the success Dance for PD and the Mark Morris Dance Group have seen by successfully engaging a large national health insurer to support delivery of their "Let's Move" dance curriculum, there are few followers from the national health plan community. And despite some local successes in scaling up social prescribing around the country, a more national movement is only in preliminary stages.

For all these reasons, I was genuinely excited when I learned that OSW set out to achieve impact and transformation via partnerships. The YMCAs have emerged as that mission-aligned partner. And I could not have been more delighted to learn that one of those leading partners was YMCA of the North, right here in Minnesota.

That didn't surprise me. I'd worked with CEO Glen Gunderson and the YMCA of the North health and wellness team around 2017, when Heart of Dance cofounder Andrea Mirenda and I introduced our Dance for Life senior curriculum to several of their Y facilities. My friend and Y board member Wendy Dayton generously funded the popular partner dance classes. Wendy has long supported the role of dance and arts in health and wellness.

So how did OSW link up with YMCA of the North? Because their activities were aligned.

When the general field of health coaching moved toward certification by the National Board for Health and Wellness Coaching, OSW pivoted to hire board-certified coaches. But they soon realized that certified coaches weren't always representative of the population. So in 2022, OSW launched its own Community as Medicine board-approved health coach training program. This not only met certification standards but also focused on cultural humility, trauma-informed health coaching, and group health coaching.

Meanwhile, YMCA of the North was also focused on building a certified health coaching program. "The health coach plays a crucial role in how YMCAs support community health and well-being by expanding the conversation from merely physical health to all aspects of a person's life—mind, body, spirit, and community," said Sally St. John, former vice president of Wellbeing Integration at YMCA of the North.

YMCA of the North published a request for proposals to find a training partner who would train thirty health coaches who identified as multicultural or a person of color. "We received over one hundred proposals, and OSW stood apart from all the rest because of our shared vision for health equity," said Sally.

"We were so lucky that Open Source Wellness rose to the top, based on the ways that we were training people to work with underserved and marginalized populations," Liz recalled. "So Y of the North sends us five people from their community each year, and we train them."

Shortly thereafter, OSW sought to create a Community as Medicine Learning Collaborative with YMCAs across the country. The goal was to build equity-centered group health coaching in partnership with local clinical health care. They issued a competitive application. YMCA of the North was selected, along with other large well-established peers: YMCA of San Diego County and YMCA of Metro Denver. They will expand that YMCA cohort in 2025.

"The idea," Liz explained, "was to spend a year not only training health coaches to deliver Community as Medicine but helping their teams figure out financial sustainability, analytics and evaluation, sustainable-equity-centered program design, and all the pieces that have to be in place for a program to be sustainable."

That includes building organizational support and readiness

and strong referral pathways. Sally's hope is that health coaching and Community as Medicine will be a pivotal solution for YMCAs to play a stronger role in improving access to lifestyle medicine and reducing chronic conditions in marginalized communities.

The partnership was a strong fit for Glen and his YMCA of the North team. "I've been particularly passionate about well-being for a long time," he said. "I've spent my whole career trying to move people to healthier places and whole-person places. There has been a perception in the community for generations that the YMCA is in the swim and gym and camp business. In reality, we're in the spirit, mind, body, and community business. If we were to move our health system upstream to focus on whole-person well-being, whole-person care, and whole-community care, we could have a demonstrative impact on the cost of care and access to care. We create a model where we care for people in keeping them well versus care for people when disease becomes manifest."

Glen notes that the Y is committed to moving from a "place-based" model to a "place-plus-platform-plus-programs" model. That includes strong digital content and platform delivery. That fits with the Y's strong equity leadership lens.

"How do we become more accessible?" Glen asks. "How do we break down barriers? As Liz noted, most of our health system has been designed for those who already have access to the system. And ultimately, can we play a role in solving what I would call the mental health tsunami that's really cutting across all segments of our population?"

According to Jennifer Menk, then executive director of the Douglas Dayton Y in downtown Minneapolis (named for Wendy Dayton's deceased husband), the dance and movement classes have been very popular, including their own version of Pedaling for Parkinson's.

"These communities were so much more than the movement," Jennifer said. "It was as much about the connection. It was about the belonging that those groups felt. And it was not only for the clients we were serving, but we started creating opportunities for the caretakers to do other things at the same time."

The key is getting enough grant funding to make these sessions part of the Y's complimentary offerings.

"We may or may not recruit enough grant funding," Glen said. "But if the health system is starting to move toward reimbursement of these kinds of activities, then how do we find our way into that pathway? The answer to that question will be a big part of the sustainability of YMCAs going forward, much less the sustainability of these programs."

That's why the YMCA of the North team was excited to launch its first Community as Medicine group in February 2025, after months of preparation. Their lead, Director of Health and Wellbeing Coaching Tim Klein, built a new clinical partnership with Herself Health, a primary care office in the Twin Cities for women sixty-five and older. They created an all-women Community as Medicine group for those who receive primary care from this network and who've been prescribed into the program by their doctors. They are prescribed for twelve weeks to participate either on site at the Y or virtually. The idea is that the participants will build relationships and enjoy the benefits of the Y's offerings, stimulating a longer-term relationship for the future.

"For me, the win is that we've helped create a bridge via this partnership," Liz said. "We've built an on-ramp to potentially a lifetime of membership and self-efficacy in their fitness and well-being journeys. This is getting people in the doors who didn't wake up one day and say, 'I want to join the Y.'"

Tim Klein also built a second clinical partnership with M Health Fairview, a large federally qualified health center based at the University of Minnesota. That Community as Medicine group will also begin in 2025.

Glen especially appreciates how Liz and her OSW team are helping the Y grow its capabilities around how to integrate with the health care system.

"They help us think through the ability to tap into the health care system," Glen said, "where we can be reimbursed over time for some of these services—which we think is a really important element to sustainability."

All good. But even better, the YMCAs present a robust opportunity of scale with a footprint of three thousand facilities serving twelve thousand communities. It's the longest-standing nonprofit in the history of the world.

The interests of OSW and the YMCA around spirit, mind, body, and community seem perfectly aligned. So how do we grow opportunities like Community as Medicine and other forms of social prescribing into the broader context of community-based whole-person health and well-being?

Glen and his team might just have a plan.

Up Next: Community-Based Whole-Person Health and Well-Being

Glen is helping to lead a regional and national effort to create a "well-being network" of the largest Ys in the country. In 2025, he began convenings with the next six largest Ys, with the hope of eventually expanding that network to the top twenty or twenty-five metropolitan service areas—or more.

"At that point," he said, "we think there'll be a brand within a brand, to the extent that the whole of the US-wide movement will want to grab hold."

Such an ambitious objective couldn't happen without aligned philanthropic partners committed to community well-being. That partner is the George Family Foundation, based in Minnesota and cochaired by Penny George, a leader in the national movement toward whole-person health and well-being for more than two decades.

The partnership between the George Family Foundation and the Y had started years before, in 2018, when the foundation created the first-of-its-kind George Wellbeing Center at the Dayton Y in downtown Minneapolis. The center was created as a space to foster community and self-care and to offer holistic healing practices that reduce stress and improve health outcomes, including meditation training, acupuncture, group mind-body classes, and other modalities.

The center came about because the George Family Foundation mission almost perfectly aligned with the Y's mission. The George Family Foundation seeks to foster wholeness in mind, body, spirit, and community by developing authentic leaders and by supporting transformative programs serving the common good. This is remarkably similar to the vision of the YMCA of the North, as an organization in the mind, body, spirit, and community business.

According to Penny, the concept of the George Wellbeing Center arose over time, as the foundation's work with Minnesota wellness pioneers yielded a consensus that community-facing organizations would get more traction.

"A lot of the ideas we were talking about related to lifestyle," Penny said. "They could be better offered outside of a health system than within one because people come into a health care system looking for a pill."

Penny also draws on her experience as a consulting psychologist and breast cancer survivor. She believes that people are connected in mind, body, and spirit with immense self-healing capacities and that we can be empowered to be the primary agent of our own health.

Former YMCA of the North vice president Sally St. John was integral to creation of the center. She explained, "The George Wellbeing Center was offering something the community was looking for: complementary healing in a trusted community-based setting. Once participants engaged with the George Wellbeing Center, the response was so strong that we needed to respond to the need and decided to offer these modalities system wide and to overhaul its mission to make whole-person health and well-being pervasive and centric to everything we do at the Y."

Even summer camps now involve nutrition and mindfulness among other aspects. And today, the health coaches trained by OSW work out of the George Wellbeing Center both in-person and virtually to improve access to care.

"Mind, body, spirit is what the Y is *about*, but community is what they *do*," Penny said. "It seems like people feel like no matter who they are, they belong there. And the fact that the Y makes their services accessible in a private way, where financial need is not an issue, is pretty remarkable. People trust the Y. By empowering the Y to do things that they already want to do, we're making optimal health accessible to more and more people in an environment in which they feel empowered and safe. I love that," she added.

Yes, the Y is all about community. And now it's time to scale up. The first step is to scale up that "well-being network" to the larger YMCA institutional network across the country. Sean Malone, president of the George Family Foundation, is excited about the possibilities.

"I think what Glen and his team are doing at Y of the North is extraordinary," Sean said. "What's really exciting is that this is so clearly the future, not just for the Ys but for communities where other key Ys have stepped in. So now there's a formal network of Ys saying this is fundamental to who we are."

The George Family Foundation was motivated to make a significant additional investment in the YMCA of the North to enhance their local offerings and to make their community-based whole-person health and well-being vision an institution-wide, system-wide transformation. That includes underwriting convenings of the leading Ys around the country to facilitate collaboration and shared practices, so each Y doesn't have to reinvent the wheel.

For example, YMCA of the North has been ramping up significant digital tools that can be shared with other Ys as well as in communities such as senior living, corporate offices, hotels, and apartment complexes. Their Virtual Y streaming platform of over eight thousand experiences integrates holistic health and well-being content into daily life. They're also sharing the benefits of health coaching and OSW partnership with other Ys. In addition, the foundation is investing in Y leaders by sponsoring them for an intensive week-long curriculum of authentic leadership development, based on the philosophy Bill George developed in *True North: Emerging Leader Edition* and his multiple other books.

Scaling up and offering leadership training to the YMCA network is a great start, but embedding these innovations even further into community is much better. So, can we scale up change beyond the footprint of YMCAs? Can partnerships like the one between the George Family Foundation and YMCA of the North be the catalyst for greater change?

And here's another million-dollar question: Is there any way our national medical system can become community based?

"The foundation and the movement haven't given up on how to transform medical systems," Sean said. "Medical systems are transactional. They have financial incentives that only compensate medical systems for prescriptions and procedures. At the end of the day, medical systems are only going to change if individuals change what they look at as being health. And they're going to find that not in the medical system—that never brings it up—but in their community."

"Empowering patients is a big part of what we want to see happen," Penny said. "When the medical systems see how much better patients do with Western medicine if they're also doing a lot more around their own lifestyle, our hope is that they'll begin to partner in some formal way so that we get people empowered. And by offering these things at the Y, we have greater access to the things that make optimum health more realistic."

That's a big vision. It also aligns with OSW's vision. We need all these pathways to make community-based whole-person wellness happen. It's all about community and empowering individuals to take charge of their own health.

"What if we made the healthy thing the easy thing?" asked

Liz of OSW. "What if Community as Medicine were as easy to walk into as a McDonald's on a Tuesday night? I know that's aspirational. But every human being needs these basics: 'Move, Nourish, Connect, and Be.' It's not rocket science. And it's not even that expensive."

Clearly, this vision of community-based whole-person wellness goes well beyond dance classes or even the arts. But just imagine how the doors would open for all of us if community-based whole-person health and well-being was the "easy thing."

We can do this. It's about creating a new social structure that makes it easy for all of us to meet our basic human needs. And in the end, the most powerful influencer is YOU!

So here's your Call to Action:

- Educate your policymakers. Most of them are likely not even aware of these community-based health and wellness possibilities. The more the public steps up, the more policymakers will respond and look for innovative community-based partnerships within state and local governments.
- Let your health provider know this is important to you. Educate your physician and network provider about recent breakthroughs in community-based health and well-being, such as social prescribing and Community as Medicine. If more patients request these options, then more providers will ask for and perhaps help create these opportunities with the medical facilities and health plans that employ or contract with them.
- Educate your insurance provider. Request these options at your next enrollment fair.
- Let your favorite arts organization know about social prescribing and Community as Medicine. Large arts organizations have influence in the community with their patrons. They have influence with their health care partners.
- Raise public awareness in traditional media, social media, and public venues. Spread the word about the benefits of

community-based whole-person health and well-being and its various forms.

- Support community organizations such as YMCA of the North and others that are taking the leap into these new venues on your behalf. Support the "brand within a brand" your community YMCA is building.
- Support medical entities such as Herself Health, M Health Fairview, and other entities working with Community as Medicine groups. Let them know you appreciate their leadership.
- Let philanthropic organizations and foundations like the George Family Foundation know that their community-based whole-person health and well-being work is meaningful to you.
- Advocate for funding for research to grow data on the effectiveness of these community-based options.
- Advocate for community-based whole-person health and well-being options to be available for all members of community, not just for those who already have access to health care.

It won't be easy. Change takes time. Our health care system is complicated. It'll take persistence and, yes, resilience.

This Call to Action gives new meaning to the Dance of Resilience. This book is about building personal resilience within each of us through partner dance. That's important. But raising our voices together will help create opportunities for all of us. That's a Community of Resilience.

It's the power of one . . . plus one . . . plus one.

It's the power of community.

Dance on!

Acknowledgments

For me, dance has always been about community. The people in that community wrapped their arms around me as this book took shape over five years. I am grateful for every person who gave me a word of encouragement, counsel, and critique. That's too many people to name, but you know who you are.

First, thank you to the magicians who helped make this book possible. For editing, I turned to Angela Wiechmann of A. M. W. Editing, LLC. Her quality editing on my first book, *Zero Chance of Passage*, was instrumental to its success. For this book, her developmental focus over time included gentle coaching as well as editing. She greatly improved the manuscript. I'm also indebted to Brooke Warner, publisher of She Writes Press, for her patience and for making this book possible with the help of project manager Shannon Green.

Then there is my assistant, Maria Wesserle, upon whom I relied more and more during the process. She educated me on everything from setting up Zoom meetings, making interview transcripts, managing dozens of electronic consents, organizing photos, conducting research, and generally keeping me on track. Patience is her virtue too.

My kitchen cabinet of dancers was invaluable. First my connectors: Nathan Daniels Hawes, my former dance instructor and dear friend, who helped me connect to others in the national dance world. Then there's dance judge Maria Hansen of Dance Vision Foundation who supported me countless times because she lives the mission of the book. And David Leventhal of Dance for PD in New York, who educated me not only on the Dance for PD story but also on the emerging national scene in research, social prescribing, and community health and well-being.

Next are my advisors: Dancers and condo neighbors Lorie Hurst, C. J. Hurst, and Marlene Kapitan Nelson (Marlene also assisted with research). Also fellow dance students Angie Star, Maryann Kudalis, Alicia Keyes, Elizabeth Dickinson, Dan Browning, and Dennis Yelkin, my social dance partner. Photographer and author Craig Blacklock as well. Thank you all for your feedback, encouragement, and wonderful ideas.

Next are the dancer storytellers who took time to share their authentic stories and their vulnerabilities with the world. I'll list them here according to their order of appearance in the book, and I'll note the dance professionals with asterisks: Dennis Yelkin; Roger and Melinda Martin; Jim Carter and Andrea Kuzel*; Dr. Paul Cederberg and Meghan Afonkin*; Lisa Davis and Markus Cannon*; Regina Kim; Greta Anderson Culkins; Cindy Snyder and Scott Anderson*; Maryann Kudalis and Dr. John Carlson; Dan Browning and my political mentor Mike Berman; Peter and Seth Westlake; Angela Calabria and daughter Alissa Quinn; Loisa Donnay*; Heart of Dance participants; Nathan Daniels Hawes*; Patrick Moriarity; Art and Cheri Rolnick; Dr. Scott and Bernie Osborn; Lorie and C. J. Hurst; Elena* and Gene* Bersten; Alex Tecza*; Kato Lindholm*; Heather Wudstrack*; Sarah Merz; Arun Garg; Choua Lee; Dr. Don DeBoer*; Maria Hansen*; Esther Frances*; Michael Finney and Linda Muir*; Jessica Roeder*; and Libby Lincoln*.

The following interviewees, some of whom are dancers, also shared unique professional expertise: life coach Angela Star; Jacob Wetterling Resource Center director Alison Feigh; dance/movement therapist Michael Gardos Reid; Dr. Brad Moser MD of Twin Cities Orthopedics; physical therapist Dr. Megin Sabo John (now with Imua Physical Therapy, Maui); Social Prescribing USA cofounder Dr. Alan Siegel; Open

Source Wellness cofounder Dr. Elizabeth Markle; YMCA of the North CEO Glen Gunderson; Dayton Y (Minneapolis) Executive Director Jennifer Menk; former YMCA of the North Vice President Sally St. John (now with Open Source Wellness); George Family Foundation cochair Penny George; and George Family Foundation President Sean Malone.

The book would not have gotten its start if *Sheer Dance*, a local online magazine, hadn't agreed to publish my dance stories on a monthly basis over a period of two years. That was the genesis of the material for this book. My thanks go to editor Taylor Wall and her publication team, as well as to Nels Petersen, the connector.

I must also give a shout-out to my current dance instructors. My primary instructor is Martin Pickering of Cinema Ballroom. My technical dancing for competition has improved greatly in the three years I've danced with him, and that makes me smile. Chris (Kempainen) Inveen of Dance Mpls has been my favorite instructor for musical theater showcase solos, including *Cabaret* and *My Fair Lady*. And I have long enjoyed dancing with instructor Scott Anderson at Soul Ballroom, who somehow got me here in the first place.

And finally, the most important people in my life gave me good counsel and total support throughout the process of this book. Thanks to my sister, Helene Johnson (proofreader extraordinaire), and my sister-in-law and author, Mary Junge. And many thanks to my nondancer husband, Mike Junge, who supported me all along the way, allowing me the time and freedom to make this happen. And yes, we have kept our promises from our wedding day, over thirty years ago: I wouldn't teach Mike how to dance, and he wouldn't teach me how to golf. It's working. We're still together. And I'm loving that most of all.

Notes

Chapter 27

1. Christine Haseler, Ranulf Crooke, and Tobias Haseler, "Promoting Physical Activity to Patients," *British Medical Journal* (2019) 366: 15230.
2. Office of the Surgeon General, *Our Epidemic of Loneliness and Isolation: The U.S. Surgeon General's Advisory on the Healing Effects of Social Connection and Community* (US Department of Health and Human Services, 2023). www.hhs.gov/sites/default/files/surgeon-general-social-connection-advisory.pdf.
3. Joe Verghese et al., "Leisure Activities and the Risk of Dementia in the Elderly," *New England Journal of Medicine* (2003) 348: 2508–16.
4. Richard Powers, "Use It or Lose It: Dancing Makes You Smarter, Longer," *Stanford Dance*, July 30, 2010. https://socialdance.stanford.edu/syllabi/smarter.htm.
5. Michael Fang et al., "Lifetime Risk and Projected Burden of Dementia," *Nature Medicine* (2025). doi.org/10.1038/s41591-024-03340-9.
6. Peter Lovatt, *The Dance Cure* (Octopus, 2020), 95.

Chapter 34

1. "The NeuroArts Blueprint Initiative," *NeuroArts Blueprint: Advancing the Science of Arts, Health and Wellbeing*, accessed February 28, 2025. www.neuroartsblueprint.org.

2. Constantina Theofanopoulou, PhD, "Neurobiology of Dance," accessed February 28, 2025. www.constantinatheo-fanopoulou.com.

Chapter 35

1. Rachel Chen, "Why Some Doctors Are Prescribing Ballroom Dance or a Day at the Museum," *Time*, June 15, 2022. time.com/6187850/social-prescriptions-improve-health.
2. "Unconventional Approach to Geriatric Complaints Appears to Decrease Emergency Visits and Symptoms," *Cleveland Clinic Consult QD*, January 31, 2023. consultqd.clevelandclinic.org/unconventional-approach-to-geriatric-complaints-appears-to-decrease-emergency-visits-and-symptoms.
3. Bethann Steiner, "Introducing the First Statewide Social Prescribing Solution in the U.S.," Mass Cultural Council, June 27, 2024. massculturalcouncil.org/blog/introducing-the-first-statewide-social-prescribing-solution-in-the-u-s.
4. Robin Wander, "Arts-Based Social Prescribing Comes to Stanford," *Stanford Report*, November 27, 2023. news.stanford.edu/stories/2023/11/arts-based-social-prescribing-comes-stanford.
5. Angela Thomas, "NJPAC receives unprecedented grant from the National Endowment for the Arts (NEA)," *NJPAC*, May 16, 2024. www.njpac.org/press/njpac-receives-unprecedented-grant-from-the-national-endowment-for-the-arts-nea.

Chapter 36

1. Elizabeth Markle, "Community as Medicine," TEDx Cherry Creek Women, Denver, November 17, 2023, 18 minutes. www.youtube.com/watch?v=cyNLd746V_o.
2. "Impact and Outcomes," *Open Source Wellness*, accessed March 3, 2025. www.opensourcewellness.org/outcomes.
3. Elizabeth Markle, "Community as Medicine," TEDx Cherry Creek Women, Denver, November 17, 2023, 18 minutes. www.youtube.com/watch?v=cyNLd746V_o.

Photo Credits

Page 107
Chapter 2, All photos courtesy of author

Page 108
Chapter 2, Photo courtesy of author

Page 109
Chapter 3, Both photos by Ryan Kenner Photography

Page 110
Chapter 4, Photo courtesy of Roger and Melinda Martin
and family
Chapter 5, Photo by Kristian Gaasland
Chapter 6, Photo courtesy of Dr. Paul Cederberg

Page 111
Chapter 7, Photo by Charles Ryder Photography
Chapter 8, Photo courtesy of Regina Kim

Page 112
Chapter 11, Photo by Charles Ryder Photography
Chapter 12, Photo courtesy of Dr. John Carlson
Chapter 13, Mike Berman: Photo courtesy of author
Chapter 13, Dan Browning: Photo courtesy of Dan Browning

Page 113
Chapter 14, Both photos courtesy of Pete Westlake
Chapter 15, Photo by Joan Heffler Photography

Page 114
Chapter 16, All photos by C. J. Hurst

Page 163
Chapter 18, Both photos courtesy of author

Page 164
Chapter 19, Author with three dance instructors:
With Gordon Bratt: Photo by Ryan Kenner Photography
With Martin Pickering: Photo by Maurice Algarra/MemMaurice
    Photography
With Scott Anderson: Photo by Charles Ryder Photography

Page 165
Chapter 20, Scott and Bernie Osborn: Photo by Ryan Kenner
    Photography
Chapter 20, Art and Cheri Rolnick: Photo courtesy of Rolnicks
Chapter 21, Photo by Lucas Erlandson

Page 166
Chapter 22, Gene and Elena Bersten (at USDC): Photo by
    Charles Ryder Photography
Chapter 22: Two Bersten family photos: courtesy of
    Bersten family

Page 167
Chapter 23, Girls in Blue: Photo by Charles Ryder Photography
Chapter 23, Alex and Kato: Photo by Natalie Fiol Photography
Chapter 24, Photo courtesy of Cheu and Choua Lee
Chapter 25, Photo by Rebecca Abas

Page 168

Chapter 26, Photo by Alex Gilman Photography

Chapter 28, Dementia dance class: Photo by Luiz C. Ribeiro Photography

Chapter 28, Wayne and Donna Eng: Photo by Siamak Arghami

Chapter 28, Maria Hansen: Photo courtesy of Maria Hansen

Page 169

Chapter 29, Photo by Chris Dudas

Chapter 30, Woman (front) in purple: Photo by Amber Star Merkens, courtesy of Dance for PD®/Mark Morris Dance Group

Chapter 30, Large group: Photo by Eddie Marritz, courtesy of Dance for PD®/Mark Morris Dance Group

Chapter 32, Photo courtesy of Michael Gardos Reid

Page 170

Chapter 33, Dr. Brad Moser: Photo courtesy of Dr. Brad Moser

Chapter 33, Dr. Megin Sabo John: Photo courtesy of Dr. Megin John

Chapter 35, Photo courtesy of Dr. Alan Siegel

Chapter 36, Photo courtesy of Dr. Elizabeth (Liz) Markle

Index

About the Author

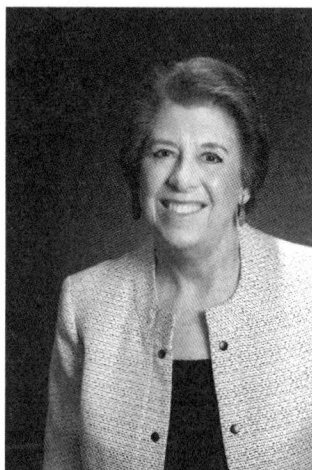

Author Photo by Rory Thomas O'Neill

E mber Reichgott Junge is the unlikely author of *The Dance
of Resilience*. She's a former eighteen-year Minnesota state
senator, a nearly fifty-year business and nonprofit attorney and
consultant, a long-time television political analyst, and a former
executive of Lutheran Social Service of Minnesota.

She's an amateur ballroom dancer who walked into a dance
studio at the age of thirty-five for one reason: to find a husband.
She found one, but he doesn't dance. Dance changed *her*.

Ember is also a former journalist. During the pandemic, she
started interviewing people who had transformed their lives
through partner dance. The dancers' passion and resilience
shone through the interviews. Ember wanted others to learn
about these experiences and the benefits of partner dance—
hence, the authentic and personal stories within the book.

As a policy advocate, Ember also interviewed leaders in various health fields to shine a light on the physical, social, mental, and emotional benefits of dance and to make a case for including dance and the arts in the larger health care system.

Ember is cofounder of Heart of Dance, a Minnesota nonprofit created in 2015 to bring the benefits of dance to fifth and eighth graders in schools and to seniors in community. She is an alumna of the international musical cast of Up with People (1971–72).

This is Ember's second book. Her first book, *Zero Chance of Passage: The Pioneering Charter School Story*, is a historical memoir of her roller-coaster journey as senate author of the first charter school law in the nation. In 2013, her book won Grand Prize for the Writer's Digest Self-Published Book Awards, among other awards. It was cited as an expert resource in a 2025 US Supreme Court case.

Ember lives in Minneapolis and is a graduate of St. Olaf College, Duke University Law School, and the University of St. Thomas MBA program. She is married to retired longtime McLeod County Attorney Michael Junge, who lives in Hutchinson. They commute between their homes with their miniature schnauzer, Maya.